Walking Atlanta

Sara Hines Martin

 Endorsed by the American Volkssport Association

GUILFORD, CONNECTICUT
FALCON® An imprint of The Globe Pequot Press

𝘈FALCONGUIDE®

Copyright © 2002 by The Globe Pequot Press

Falcon and FalconGuide are registered trademarks of The Globe Pequot Press.

Cover photo by Henryk Kaiser/Index Stock
Maps by Moore Creative Designs
All photos by the author unless otherwise noted.

Library of Congress Cataloging-in-Publication Data
Martin, Sara Hines, 1933–
     Walking Atlanta / Sara Hines Martin.
          p. cm.
     Includes index.
     ISBN 0-7627-1015-2
     1. Atlanta (Ga.)—Tours. 2. Walking—Georgia—Atlanta—
Guidebooks. 3. Historic sites—Georgia—Atlanta—Guidebooks. I.
Title.
F294.A83 M37 2001
917.58'2310444—dc21   2001053207

Manufactured in the United States of America
First Edition/First Printing

Contents

The Walks

Science and Natural History

Historic Mountain Parks

Beyond Atlanta

Acknowledgments

I have depended upon many helpful people to secure the information needed for this book. Ren and Helen Davis's book served as a valuable guide. Enthusiastic Mary Ann Hearn at the Atlanta Convention and Visitors Bureau gave me a great deal of help. Emily Kleine at the Atlanta Preservation Center provided information about historic districts, and the volunteers who led the walks were passionate about their city. Robin Reid at Clark-Atlanta University helped me tour the Atlanta University Center, and Terrance Watkins showed me around Morris Brown College. Alix Hintze took me on a guided tour of the Atlanta Botanical Garden, and Alice Richards took me on a tour of the nature trail at Stone Mountain. David Funderburk took me on two guided walks on the Fernbank Science Center trail. Don Bender walked with me on the Freedom Path. Retha Stephens, Park Ranger at Kennesaw Mountain National Battlefield Park, gave me information about the trail and allowed me to copy precious historic photographs. Harold Harmon, volunteer reenactor, gave me details about the battles there. Lisa Littlefield gave me a tour of the Atlanta History Museum and free tickets to the historic houses there. Horticulturist Sue Vroorman gave me helpful printed material on the Swan Woods Trail. Dr. Laura Dorsey gave me the same about the Peace Garden on the trail. Megan Winokur gave me a tour through Zoo Atlanta, and Pauline Smith, Director, hosted me at the Cyclorama. Alison Tyrer helped me at the Margaret Mitchell House & Museum. David Arnold, Public Relations Director at Georgia Institute of Technology, drove me around the campus. Elayne Hunter and Michael Jardine assisted me at the Outdoor Activity Center. Zach Pfeiffer prepared the information and the trail markers at

Kennesaw National Battlefield Park for a 1987 Eagle Scout project in Marietta, Georgia.

I'm also grateful to the friends who went on the walks with me, serving as extra eyes and ears. While I was encumbered with notebook, pen, camera, and guidebook, they helped me by telling me where I was (when I was standing right under a street sign).

Map Legend

Walk Route		River or Stream	
Streets and Roads		Lake or Pond	
Start/Finish of Loop Walk	S/F	Interstate	75
Parking Area	P	U.S. Highway	78
Building		Railroad	+++++++
Church or Cathedral	†	Steps	
Restrooms, Male and Female		Parkland	
Accessible Facility/Trail		Overlook	
Dining Facilities			N
Playground		Map Orientation	
Ballfield		Scale of Distance	0 0.5 1
			Mile

Atlanta Overview Map

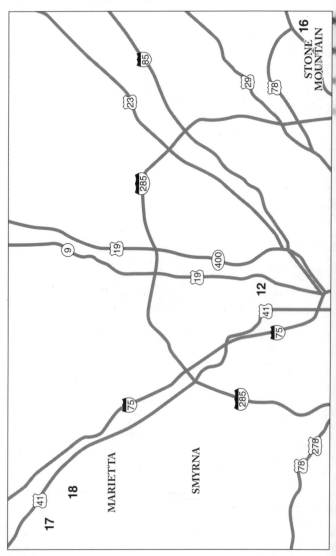

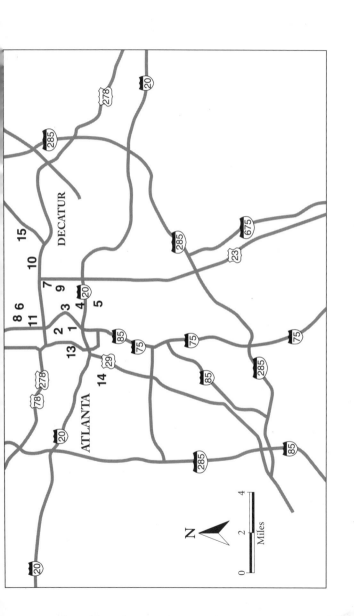

Foreword

For more than twenty years, Falcon has guided millions of people to America's wild outside, showing them where to paddle, hike, bike, bird, fish, climb, and drive. With this walking series we at Falcon ask you to try something just as adventurous. We invite you to experience this country from its sidewalks, not its back roads, and to stroll through some of America's most interesting cities.

In their haste to get where they are going, travelers often bypass this country's cities, and in the process, they miss the historic and scenic treasures hidden among the bricks. Many people seek spectacular scenery and beautiful settings on top of the mountains, along the rivers, and in the woods. While nothing can replace the serenity and inspiration of America's natural wonders, we should not overlook the beauty of the urban landscape.

The steel and glass of municipal mountains reflect the sunlight and make people feel small in the shadows. Birds sing in city parks, water burbles in the fountains, and along the sidewalks walkers can still see abundant wildlife—their fellow humans.

Falcon's many outdoor guidebooks have encouraged people not only to explore and enjoy America's natural beauty but also to preserve and protect it. Our cities are equally meant to be enjoyed and explored, and their irreplaceable treasures need care and protection.

When travelers and walkers want to explore something that is inspirational and beautiful, we hope they will lace up their walking shoes and point their feet toward one of this country's many cities. For there, along the walkways, they are sure to discover the excitement, history, beauty, and charm of urban America.

—*The Editors*

Preface: Come Walk Atlanta

Atlanta novelist Anne Rivers Siddons observes, "No city in America, perhaps, spans so many eras of history so gracefully." Nature has also blessed the city. Atlanta—"the city of trees"—sits atop a 1,000-foot ridge in the southern Piedmont. Its mild climate and its 5,000 miles of street-tree canopy permit walking year-round.

Atlanta offers miles of walking paths and hiking trails to those who want to "hoof it." It also offers sites for people with varied interests. Experience its Civil War history. As the home of Margaret Mitchell, the city attracts *Gone With the Wind* fans. The cradle of the Civil Rights movement has the home of Martin Luther King Jr., and the Center for Nonviolent Social Change.

You will visit outstanding museums and see beautiful historic churches. Visit the world-class Botanical Garden and nature's masterwork, Stone Mountain. Sample superb offerings of famous Southern foods, from fried chicken and hot biscuits to grits, barbecue, and pecan pie.

Walkers who want to pound dirt instead of pavement can head to the aesthetically pleasing, clean, and safe parks. In spring dogwood blossoms rival peaches as the city's icon in the peach state.

If business brings you here, let *Walking Atlanta* help you unwind at day's end. If vacation brings you here, get a close-up view of this popular destination. If you're a resident, *Walking Atlanta* will give your visitors a taste of the city's special offerings. From the heart of downtown, visitors can reach Atlanta's attractions, entertainment venues, restaurants, and neighborhoods, all within a short ride by cab, bus, or rail.

From the Southeast's most outstanding zoo to the historic districts, this city invites everyone to walk, explore, and enjoy.

To appreciate Atlanta's present, experience its past. From its role in the Civil War to its hosting of the 1996 Centennial Olympic Games, Atlanta promises learning and entertainment for everyone.

How to Use this Guide

Walking the streets and boulevards of a city can take you into its heart and give you a feel for its pulse and personality. From the sidewalk looking up, you can appreciate its architecture. From the sidewalk peeking in, you can find the quaint shops, local museums, and great eateries that give a city its charm and personality. From its nature paths you can smell the flowers, glimpse the wildlife, gaze at a lake, or hear a creek gurgle. Only by walking can you get close enough to read the historical plaques and watch the people. When you walk a city, you get it all—adventure, scenery, local color, good exercise, and fun.

We have designed this book so that you can easily find the walks that match your interests, time, and energy level. The Trip Planner is the first place you should look when deciding on a walk. This table will give you the basic information—a walk's distance, the estimated walking time, and the difficulty. The pictures or icons in the table also tell you specific things about the walk:

Every walk has something of interest, but this icon tells you that the route will have particular appeal to the shutterbug. So bring your camera. You will have great views of the city or the surrounding area, and you are likely to get some wonderful scenic shots.

Somewhere along the route you will have the chance to get food or a beverage. You will have to glance through the walk description to determine where and what kind of food and beverages are available. Walks that do not have the food icon probably are along nature trails or in noncommercial areas of the city.

During your walk you will have the chance to shop. More detailed descriptions of the types of stores you will find can be found in the actual walk description.

This walk features something kids will enjoy seeing or doing—a park, zoo, museum, or play equipment. In most cases the walks that carry this icon are short and follow an easy, fairly level path. You know your young walking companions best. If your children are patient walkers who do not tire easily, then feel free to choose walks that are longer and harder. In fact, depending on a child's age and energy, most children can do any of the walks in this book. The icon notes only those walks we think they will especially enjoy.

Your path will take you primarily through urban areas. Buildings, small city parks, and paved paths are what you will see and pass.

You will pass through a large park or walk in a natural setting where you can see and enjoy nature.

The wheelchair icon means that the path is fully accessible. This walk would be easy for someone pushing a wheelchair or stroller. We have made every attempt to follow a high standard for accessibility. The icon means there are curb cuts or ramps along the entire route, plus a wheelchair-accessible bathroom somewhere along the way. The path is mostly or entirely paved, and ramps and unpaved surfaces are clearly described. If you use a wheelchair and have the ability to negotiate curbs and dirt paths or to wheel for longer distances and on uneven surfaces, you may want to skim the directions for the walks that do not carry this symbol. You may find other walks you will enjoy. If in doubt, read the full text of the walk or call the contact source for guidance.

At the start of each walk description, you will find specific information describing the route and what you can expect on your walk:

General location: Here you will get the walk's general location in the city or within a specific area.

Special attractions: Look here to find the specific things you will pass. If this walk has museums, historic homes, restaurants, or wildlife, it will be noted here.

Difficulty rating: For this book we have selected walking routes that an average person in reasonable health can complete easily. In most cases you will be walking on flat surfaces with few, if any, hills. Your path will most likely be a maintained surface of concrete, asphalt, wood, or packed dirt. It will be easy to follow, and you will be only a block or so from a phone, other people, or businesses. If the walk is less than a mile, you may be able to walk comfortably in street shoes. If you are in doubt about whether you can manage a particular walk, read the description carefully or call the listed contact for more information.

Distance: This gives the total distance of the walk.

Estimated time: The time allotted for each walk is based on walking time only, which we have calculated at about 30 minutes per mile, a slow pace. Most people have no trouble walking a mile in half an hour, and people with some walking experience often walk a 20-minute mile. If the walk includes museums, shops, or restaurants, you may want to add sightseeing time to the estimate.

Services: Here you will find out if such things as rest rooms, parking, refreshments, or information centers are available and where you are likely to find them.

Restrictions: The most often noted restriction is pets, which almost always have to be leashed in a city. Most cities also have strict "pooper-scooper" laws, and they enforce them. But restrictions may also include the hours or days a museum or business is open, age requirements, or whether you can ride a bike on the path. If there is something you cannot do on this walk, it will be noted here.

For more information: Each walk includes at least one contact source for you to call for more information. If an agency or business is named as a contact, you will find its phone number and address in Appendix B. This appendix also includes contact information for any business or agency mentioned anywhere in the book.

Getting started: Here you will find specific directions to the starting point. Most walks are closed loops, which means they begin and end at the same point. Thus, you do not have to worry about finding your car or your way back to the bus stop when your walk is over.

In those cities with excellent transportation, such as Atlanta, it may be easy—and sometimes even more interesting—to end a few of your walks away from your starting point. When this happens, you will get clear directions on how to take public transportation back to your starting point.

If a walk is not a closed loop, this section will tell you when the walk ends, and you will find the exact directions back to your starting point at the end of the walk's directions.

Some downtown walks can be started at any one of several hotels the walk passes. The directions will be for the main starting point, but this section will tell you if it is possible to pick up the walk at other locations. If you are staying at a downtown hotel, it is likely that a walk passes in front of or near your hotel's entrance.

Public transportation: Many cities have excellent transportation systems; others have limited services. If it is possible to take a bus or commuter train to the walk's starting point, you will find the bus or train noted here. You may also find some information about where the bus or train stops.

Overview: Every part of a city has a story. Here is where you will find the story or stories about the people, neighborhoods, and history connected to your walk.

Trip Planner

the walks

Walk name	Difficulty	Distance (miles)	Time	🚋	🏢	🌼	🧺	🛍	🍴	📷
Historic Downtown										
1 Underground Atlanta	Easy	0.8 mile	25 minutes	✓	✓					✓
2 Five Points and Historic Downtown	Easy	1 mile	30 minutes	✓	✓			✓	✓	✓
3 Sweet Auburn/Martin Luther King Jr. Historic Site and Preservation District	Easy	2.3 miles	70 minutes	✓	✓			✓	✓	✓
Atlanta's Open Spaces										
4 Historic Oakland Cemetery	Easy	1.5 miles	45 minutes	✓		✓	✓	✓	✓	✓
5 Grant Park: Zoo Atlanta	Easy	0.8 mile	30 minutes	✓		✓	✓	✓	✓	✓
6 Piedmont Park and Atlanta Botanical Garden	Easy	1.4 miles	45 minutes	✓		✓	✓			✓
7 Freedom Path	Easy	0.8 mile	20 minutes	✓		✓	✓	✓	✓	✓
8 Freedom Path	Easy	2.4 miles	70 minutes			✓	✓			✓
Historic Neighborhoods										
8 Ansley Park	Easy	1 mile	30 minutes		✓	✓	✓	✓	✓	✓
9 Inman Park	Easy	1.6 miles	45 minutes		✓	✓	✓	✓	✓	✓
10 Druid Hills	Easy	1.3 miles	40 minutes		✓	✓	✓			✓

	Difficulty	Distance	Time	Wheelchair access	City setting	Nature setting	Good for kids	Shopping	Food	Bring Camera
Beyond Downtown										
11 Midtown	Easy	3.6 miles	2 hours		✓			✓	✓	✓
12 The Atlanta History Center	Easy	0.5 mile	15 minutes		✓		✓	✓	✓	✓
West End										
13 Atlanta University Center	Easy	3 miles	90 minutes		✓		✓			✓
14 Outdoor Activity Center	Moderate	0.75 mile	25 minutes			✓	✓			✓
Science and Natural History										
15 Fernbank Science Center and Museum of Natural History	Easy	0.8 mile	25 minutes				✓	✓		✓
Historic Mountain Parks										
16 Stone Mountain Park	Easy	0.75 mile	20 minutes			✓		✓	✓	✓
17 Kennesaw National Battlefield Park	Difficult	2 miles	60–90 minutes			✓		✓	✓	✓
Beyond Atlanta										
18 Historic Marietta	Easy	2.3 miles	70 minutes		✓		✓	✓	✓	✓

the icons

Wheelchair access · City setting · Nature setting · Good for kids · Shopping · Food · Bring Camera

Meet Atlanta

General
County: Fulton
Time zone: Eastern
Area code: 404

Size
3.9 million people in the metro area, which covers
seven counties

Elevation
1,050 feet above sea level

Climate
Average yearly precipitation: 50 inches
Average yearly days of sunshine: 216
Average yearly snowfall: 1 inch
Average maximum temperature: 70.3 degrees F
Average minimum temperature: 51.3 degrees F

Getting there
Major highways
Interstates: I–20, I–75, I–85; I–285 encircles the
city
U.S. highways: 41 and 278
State highways: 85, 70, 154, 236, and 260
Airport service
Hartsfield Atlanta International Airport

Outdoor recreation
Golf courses: forty public, twenty private
Parks: 352 city and county parks covering 5,250 acres
Rock climbing: four sites (Allenbrook, Long Island,
The Palisades, The Zipper)

Major industries
Tourism, transportation, Coca-Cola, AT&T, Georgia Pacific, Cox Communications

Media
Television stations
ABC—Channel 2
CBS—Channel 46
Fox—Channel 5
NBC—Channel 11
PBS—Channel 8
Radio stations
WCNN 680 AM—News radio
WPCH 94.9 FM—Light rock
WABE 90.1 FM National Public Radio member —Classical/news
Newspapers
The Atlanta Journal, morning daily
The Atlanta Constitution, afternoon daily

Special annual events
(Call the Atlanta Convention and Visitor's Bureau at 404–521–6600 for updated listings.)

- January: Martin Luther King Jr. Week

- February: Southeastern Flower Show, City Hall East

- April: Easter Sunrise Services, Sweet Auburn Festival, Auburn Avenue

- May: Georgia Special Olympics State Summer Games

- June: Georgia Shakespeare Festival, June–August

- July: Black Family Reunion Celebration, Peachtree 10K Road Race, July 4

- November: *Heaven Bound,* a theatrical production at Big Bethel AME Church
- December: The Atlanta Ballet's *Nutcracker,* Festival of Trees, New Year's Eve Peach Drop

Sports Teams

The Atlanta Braves Baseball Club
    Turner Field
    755 Hank Aaron Drive, SW
    Atlanta 30315
    522–7630
    Tour Info: 614–2311
    Tickets: 577–9100

The Atlanta Falcons Football Club
    The Georgia Dome, Georgia World Congress Center
    285 Andrew Young International Boulevard, NW
    Atlanta 30313–1591
    Ticket charge line: 249–6400

The Atlanta Hawks Basketball Club
    One Philips Arena Drive, NW
    Atlanta 30335
    Tickets: 827–3865

Weather

Mother Nature has bestowed upon Atlanta four distinct seasons, yet provides delightfully mild weather. Locals call it the "golf in January factor." So regardless of the month, you will usually be comfortable while walking outdoors.

July has the highest temperatures, but prevailing westerly winds help moderate sultry Southern summers. But drink plenty of noncaffeinated, nonalcoholic fluids, and carry some with you. Wear light-colored, breathable fabrics like cotton. Wear sunblock and a hat to protect your face from the sun. Warm weather can continue through October and even into November and December!

January, the coldest month, has an average temperature of 42 degrees F and an average daily low temperature of 33 degrees. January and February each average one day of snow. Be prepared to wear a coat, hat, and gloves on some winter days.

Transportation

By car: Because of Atlanta's layout, driving can be downright confusing. Some travelers have observed that Atlanta may be the only city in the world where someone may walk around the block and never come back to the starting point. Residents as well as visitors get lost.

The city's streets grew up around Indian trails, which weave, rather than follow a grid system. The railroad also helped determine the streets' layouts, adding to the confusion. The city does not lie north and south as most others. Instead, the surveyor laid out the town parallel to the railroad, which ran northwest and southeast.

Peachtree Street is the main street of the city, and it extends north to south through the city. North Avenue and Ponce de Leon Avenue are the principal east-west streets.

Metro Atlanta includes parts of seven counties. Interstate 75 runs north and south, and Interstate 85 goes from southwest to northeast. Interstate 20 goes from west to east. None of these has a street name. You can travel the fastest way into or through the city by the interstates, and they have several exits at the major streets. All intersect Interstate 285, which circles the city.

Take heart, though. If you get lost, just stop and ask for help. Atlantans take pride in their friendliness.

Downtown has plenty of paid parking lots.

By bus: MARTA (Metropolitan Atlanta Rapid Transit Authority), Atlanta's rapid-rail and bus system, has one of the cleanest, safest, and most reliable transportation systems in the world. Many of the city's attractions are within ten minutes of downtown, and you can travel to almost all of them via MARTA.

A train leaves the airport every eight minutes from 4:34 A.M. to 1:16 A.M. Monday–Friday. Take the northbound train to the Five Points station to go to the heart of the city. You can buy tickets for $1.75 each at the airport. Call MARTA for times and schedules for the routes you need during your stay.

The north-south and east-west rail lines intersect at the Five Points station, where riders can transfer trains at no extra charge. MARTA has thirty-six stations and 150 bus routes covering the metropolitan area. Eighteen multilingual information kiosks at thirteen of its busiest rail stations provide recordings for international visitors.

All MARTA stations and rapid-rail cars are fully accessible to elders and persons with physical disabilities. In addition, special MARTA L-Vans have lifts for easy boarding and safety belts for securing wheelchairs. MARTA establishes these special routes in response to individual requests and provides door-to-door service. The one-way fare costs $3.00, and required attendants ride free. Seniors and the disabled may buy half-fare cards at the Five Points station.

By air: Millions of people pass through Hartsfield Atlanta International Airport each year. It is the world's busiest airport, and it has the world's largest passenger-terminal complex. Hartsfield employs thousands of people—making it Georgia's largest employer. With its own post office, mass-transit system, newspaper, and police and fire departments, this self-contained city never sleeps.

You may visit one of the Atlanta Convention and Visitors Bureau centers at the airport at 5000 North Terminal-PRW-West Cross Over. The bureau has a helpful staff and a wealth of information—most of it free—on places to stay and eat and things to do in the area.

Taxi service from the airport to the downtown will cost about $20 per passenger.

By train: Amtrak's *The Crescent* runs once daily through Atlanta from New Orleans to Washington, D. C., and back.

Safety

Mention a big city, and many people immediately think of safety. Some questions are frequently asked: Is it safe to walk during the day? What about at night? What areas should I avoid?

Safety should be a commonsense concern whether you are walking in a small town or a big city, but safety does not have to be your overriding concern. America's cities are enjoyable places, and if you follow some basic tips, you will find that these cities are also safe places.

Any safety mishap in a large city is likely to come from petty theft or vandalism, so the biggest tip is simple: Do not tempt thieves. Purses dangling on shoulder straps or slung over your arm, wallets peeking out of pockets, arms burdened with packages, valuables on the car seat—all of these things attract the pickpocket, purse snatcher, or thief. You look like someone who could be easily relieved of your possessions.

Do not carry a purse. Put your money in a money belt or tuck your wallet into a deep side pocket of your pants or skirt or in a fanny pack that rides over your hip bone and stomach. Lock your valuables in the trunk of your car before you park and leave for your walk. Protect your camera by wearing the strap across your chest, not just over your shoulder; better yet, put your camera in a backpack.

You also will feel safer if you remember the following:

- Be aware of your surroundings and the people near you.

- Avoid parks or other isolated places at night.

- Walk with others.

- Walk in well-lit and well-traveled areas.

- Stop and ask directions if you get lost.

The walks in this book were selected with safety in mind. None of them will take you through a bad neighborhood or into an area of the city that is known to be dangerous. So relax and enjoy your walk.

Atlanta spent $2 billion to improve its streetscapes and infrastructure for the 1996 Olympic Games. These changes make the city's parks and streets perfect for strolls or picnics.

The Downtown Improvement District's Ambassador Force, begun during the 1996 Olympic Games, has made Atlanta cleaner, safer, and more vibrant. About fifty well-trained "ambassadors" patrol downtown, helping visitors with directions and information and offering emergency assistance. They work with the Atlanta Police Department to serve in a nonconfrontational role as the APD's eyes and ears. They carry radios and report happenings on the street; when needed, they call law-enforcement personnel.

Look for the ambassadors in their white pith helmets, white shirts, aqua jackets, and navy pants with a red stripe. Just walk up and ask for help.

The Story of Atlanta

The region was occupied in the past by the Creek Indians. The War of 1812 brought the first white people to the land that is now Atlanta, most of them soldiers. Because the Creek Nation had allied with the British, American troops built two forts in the area—Fort Daniels and Fort Peachtree. These forts stood at the mouth of Peachtree Creek at the Chattahoochee River, near the Indian trading post called Standing Peachtree.

Peachtree Road—the city's first major roadway—connected the forts and the trading post. The route later became Atlanta's well-known Peachtree Street. In Buckhead it becomes Peachtree Road, and, finally, it becomes Peachtree Industrial Boulevard.

In these early days on Peachtree Street, farmers' wagon wheels often bogged down in the muddy, rutted road. Although the city's streets have changed a great deal since those days, one thing remains the same—confusion over the abundance of streets carrying "Peachtree" in their names. At present about a hundred streets in the Atlanta metropolitan area share this historic moniker. Where else but Peachtree Street would Margaret Mitchell have located Rhett and Scarlett's mansion in *Gone With the Wind?*

After the military presence the railroads took their turns shaping Atlanta's history and traffic patterns. By 1837 the railroads had entered Atlanta from all directions. The town first came to be called Terminus because so many rail lines met here. Col. Stephen Long, who chose the site for the terminus, saw a limited future for the town. He said it would be a good location for a grocery, a blacksmith shop, and a tavern, but nothing else. Fortunately his prediction was not accurate.

In 1843 the flourishing town changed its name to Marthasville, after Martha Lumpkin, the daughter of Gov. Wilson Lumpkin, who had obtained the railroad charter. But the name didn't stick, and two years later a Georgia railroad engineer proposed renaming the town Atlanta. The new name was a reference to the Western and Atlantic Railroad, which terminated in the city.

Atlanta's strength as a railroad center brought the Civil War here. Present-day Atlantans know the Civil War by several names: The War between the States, The Great Unpleasantness, The War against Northern Aggression, or The War for Southern Independence. Some people just call it The War. By any name the conflict mostly spared Atlanta until July 1864. Although the city served mainly as a hospital and relief center for Confederate soldiers, its rail and manufacturing centers were key elements in supplying the Confederate armies in the field. Consequently, Gen. William T. Sherman, commander of the Union army then moving east from Tennessee, concluded that he had to destroy the city to defeat the Confederacy.

The Battle of Atlanta started on July 22, 1864, and continued until the end of August, when Mayor James M. Calhoun surrendered the city to Sherman. The fighting destroyed more than 4,500 buildings, including schools, churches, and the state penitentiary. Two-thirds of the homes in the city were destroyed. Historians still debate whether Sherman ordered widespread burning of the city or if his soldiers simply exceeded their orders. The Confederate troops added to the conflagration when they burned their remaining supplies to keep them from falling into enemy hands. Most of the city's residents fled as the Union troops moved in.

Sherman's army left Atlanta on November 15, 1864. As his soldiers embarked on their infamous March to the Sea, they met some Atlanta citizens headed back into the city. On foot and in mule carts, they were returning to begin the process of rebuilding. Mayor Calhoun found $1.64 in the city's treasury.

Atlanta endured a harsh era of Reconstruction. Confederate money had no value. People had so little food that for three years after the war, 35,000 people around Atlanta depended on the federal government's food distribution to survive. But the city did rise again. Its citizens chose the phoenix—the mythical bird that rose from its ashes—as its symbol.

In 1877 Atlanta became Georgia's fifth—and final—state capital. By 1900 the city had become the third-largest business railhead in the country.

In May 1917 a fire destroyed more of Atlanta than Sherman's torches had. Once again the city rose like a phoenix from those ashes. The Great Depression and the enormous social upheaval of the 1950s each took a toll on the city, and each time it came back stronger. Modern Atlanta is a cosmopolitan city that boasts businesses of all types and residents from almost every country in the world. It has more restaurants, entertainment venues, and cultural attractions than any other city in the Southeast.

Atlanta has successful professional sports teams and state-of-the-art sports facilities. It has hosted some of the world's most prestigious sporting events, including Super Bowl XXVIII and several World Series. The 1996 Centennial Olympic Games drew the largest number of people at a peacetime gathering in the history of the world. More than 10,000 athletes from nearly 200 countries participated in the seventeen-day event, which brought more than two million visitors from all over the world to Atlanta. More than two-thirds of the world's population—3.5 billion people—saw the city via worldwide television coverage.

Historic Horse Swap

Atlanta began on a parcel of land that Samuel Mitchell received in a horse swap. Mitchell lived in Zebulon, Georgia, a small town 40 miles south of Terminus, the future Atlanta. He and Margaret Mitchell, author of *Gone With the Wind*, may have been distant cousins.

One night Mitchell sheltered a stranger who came to his farm. Benjamin Beckman planned to stay only a short while, but he became ill and stayed longer. When he was well enough to leave, he wanted to swap his horse for one of Mitchell's. But Mitchell thought his horse was worth more than Beckman's, and he wouldn't trade unless his visitor sweetened the pot.

In 1838 Beckman had won a plot of land in a land lottery. He offered the land—valued at $44—to Mitchell to even up the horse trade. Thus Mitchell came to own land in an area near Fort Peachtree, which would one day become the heart of Atlanta.

In the 1830s the Western and Atlantic Railroad wanted to come from Chattanooga to link up with the Central of Georgia's line coming from Savannah. The chief engineer of the Western and Atlantic Railroad decided where the end point of his railroad would fall. And guess who owned that plot of land? Sam Mitchell. In response to an appeal from a railroad official, Mitchell donated the land to Georgia in 1842.

The railroad wanted to rename Terminus "Mitchellville," but Mitchell declined the honor. He asked only that a street be named for him. You may walk on this street in Walk 1.

And just eleven days after the close of the Centennial Olympic Games, Atlanta hosted more than 3,500 athletes with disabilities from more than 120 nations during the Paralympic Games.

Atlanta's can-do spirit has led many people to proclaim it as "Capital of the New South." It is the Southeast's center for transportation, finance, retail, industry, communications, education, health care, sports, music, and culture. Atlanta's quality of life puts it among the most popular U.S. cities. Many people consider it among the nation's friendliest cities, and it is a top pick for many business travelers.

I hope the walks in this book will guide the reader to Atlanta in its many aspects: its vibrant downtown and pleasant residential neighborhoods, a bit of the city's history, and perhaps even a glimpse of its promising future.

Walk 1
Underground Atlanta

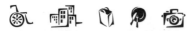

General location: Explore the heart of downtown Atlanta in a walk that takes you back to the time of the city's founding.

Special attractions: Atlanta Convention and Visitors Bureau Visitors Center, historic landmarks, Underground Atlanta, World of Coca-Cola Museum, three historic churches, Fulton County Government Center.

Difficulty rating: Fairly level with some inclines, entirely on sidewalks.

Distance: 0.8 mile.

Estimated time: 25 minutes.

Services: Restaurants and rest rooms are available in Underground Atlanta; rest rooms and soft drinks are available in World of Coca-Cola Museum; rest rooms are available in Visitors Center and in government buildings.

Underground Atlanta

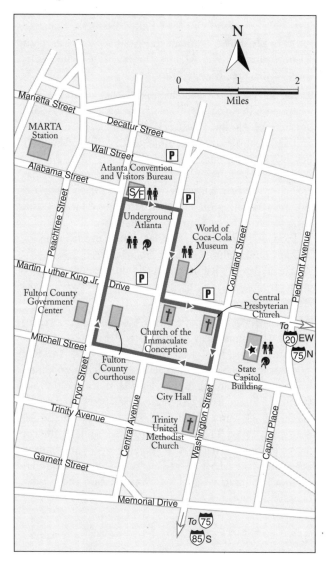

Restrictions: No dogs are allowed in Underground Atlanta. On the streets dogs must be on leashes no longer than 6 feet, and their droppings have to be picked up.

For more information: Contact the Atlanta Convention and Visitors Bureau. The Atlanta Preservation Center offers tours of this area March–November.

Getting started: This walk begins at the Visitors Center location on Pryor Street. To reach the center from I–85/75 South, take exit 246 (Butler, J. W. Dobbs), go to the second light, and turn right on Auburn. Take Auburn to Peachtree Street and go left. Turn left onto Mitchell Avenue and left onto Central to Park 90 Central, or park at one of the two lots across the street. Or you may turn left onto Washington and then left onto Martin Luther King Jr. Drive to parking lots on that street.

From I–85/75 North, take exit 248A and take the second left onto Auburn Avenue. Follow directions above.

The Atlanta Visitors Center is on the upper level of Underground Atlanta. Pick up a copy of *Walking Tour of Historic Sites and Markers* there.

Public transportation: Take MARTA from the airport. It is only a 15-minute trip to the Five Points station at 30 Alabama Street, S.W. Exit there. You may exit MARTA at a passageway to the lower level of Underground, but it is best to exit at the upper level and turn right onto Peachtree Street. Turn left to cross Peachtree Street at the corner of Alabama. Walk past the fountain on the left; then cross Pryor. The center is at 65 Alabama at the corner of Pryor and Alabama. If you are staying at a hotel on Peachtree, take MARTA at Peachtree Center station and go south. Contact MARTA for information about times, fares, and routes.

Walk 1

Overview: Underground Atlanta, Atlanta's "city beneath the city," actually has two levels. Most of Underground is on the upper level, where you find the Visitors Center. On the level below street level, you will be walking on the ground that Sam Mitchell donated. The courtyard connects with Upper Alabama Street, home of fashionable shops. Visitors can take stairs or an escalator to Lower Alabama and Lower Pryor Streets, the original streets of old Atlanta and site of old Underground.

Underground came about because of the problems the railroads caused. The trains caused clogged traffic, cinders that hurt people's eyes, and lots of noise. Between 1901 and 1929 several bridges had moved city life to the street above the original milepost. Underground exists in that tunnel created by the bridges.

In the early days Underground went by the name Humbug Square, one of the city's rougher sections. Jugglers, musicians, dancing bears, and "drummers"—snake-oil salesmen and medicine men—entertained passersby.

In 1837 Georgia caught the national railroad fever. Crews searched for the spot where a railroad could pass around the mountains. Col. L. P. Grant, an army engineer, drove a Zero Mile Marker with the inscription W&AR (the Western and Atlantic Railroad) into the ground. It marks the starting point of the railroad when Atlanta had the name Terminus. Atlanta spread outward.

Since Atlanta had become a rail hub of the region by the time of the Civil War, Gen. William T. Sherman's troops burned it. One of the first bombs of the Battle of Atlanta landed near Underground. In 1864 the troops burned the Freight Depot—shown in several *Gone With the Wind* scenes—1 block east of Underground. A replica

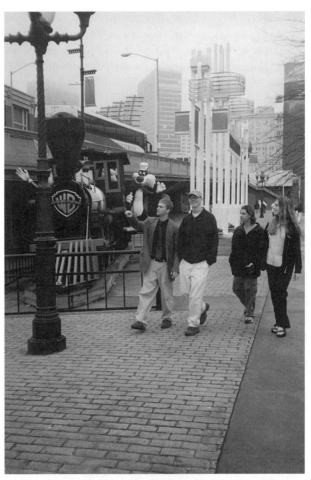

Underground Atlanta creates the ambience of the 1850s with cobble-stone streets and gaslights.

replaced the depot, which is the oldest building in downtown Atlanta, along with the Shrine of the Immaculate Conception.

Underground disappeared for many years, but in 1980 it was listed as a National Historic Site. New Underground—6 city blocks—came about in 1989. The authentic restorations of the cobblestone streets with gaslights take you back to the 1850s. At that time the shops, saloons, and cafes served people connected to the rail center.

The World of Coca-Cola Museum, across the street from Underground, may be the largest building ever erected to advertising.

You will pass historic churches, the State Capitol Building, City Hall, and the Fulton County Government Center, one of the only city-county-state government office complexes in the United States.

The Walk

➤Start at the Atlanta Visitors Center.

➤Turn left as you leave the center and walk through the courtyard. Notice the symbol of the phoenix overhead on the left.

➤As you cross Central, you may want to enter the left entrance of the parking garage at 90 Central, go through the doorway marked ZERO MILE PRECINCT POLICE, and take the elevator to the lower-level police station. There you will see the Zero Mile Marker, originally located nearby and placed at this point in 1842.

A Brew That Grew

In 1886 Atlanta pharmacist John S. Pemberton mixed a brew in his backyard. He called it "French Wine Cola, the Ideal Nerve and Tonic Stimulant." He exchanged the wine for a pinch of caffeine with the extract of cola and then mixed the syrup with water. He charged 5 cents for this drink advertised to cure hangovers, soothe queasy stomachs, and calm nerves. It also helped beat the heat in summertime. Pemberton's bookkeeper first wrote the name Coca-Cola, thinking it would sound good in ads.

Druggist Asa G. Candler had come to town with $1.75 in his pocket. Finding the new drink helpful for his own queasy stomach, he bought the formula for $2,300. He sold the syrup to soda fountains all over the country, places where people gathered originally just to talk.

Two lawyers decided to bottle the drink so that people could also take it home with them. Candler did not think much of the idea, so in 1899 he sold the bottling rights to the men for $1.00. He never bothered to collect it.

By accident another distinctive change took place in the drink itself. Instead of plain water, someone mixed in carbonated water, which people liked even better.

In 1912 an employee said, "We need a new bottle . . . which a person will recognize . . . even when he feels it in the dark." This idea led to the creation of the now-familiar bottle shape.

When Robert Woodruff became president of Coca-Cola in 1923, the company was selling almost six million drinks per day. He took the product worldwide, and when he retired thirty years later, the company was selling fifty million drinks a day.

You can see the site of Pemberton's drugstore in Walk 2 and read more about the Coca-Cola company in Walk 11.

►Walk down the stairs. You will face the 1869 depot that replaced the original. It is the oldest structure in the central city.

►At the foot of the stairs, you will pass the entrance to the lower level of Underground Atlanta on the right.

►Pass the fountain and the World of Coca-Cola pavilion on the left.

►Cross Martin Luther King Jr. Drive at the corner and turn left. The Church of the Immaculate Conception, the city's oldest religious establishment, stands on the corner. The war damaged the first building, completed in 1848. The current building, built between 1869 and 1873, has French Gothic and English High Victorian Gothic architectural elements. Gen. William T. Sherman used the church as a hospital during the occupation. In August

Of Interest

Thank Heaven for Father O'Reilly

Because of Father Thomas O'Reilly, the Shrine of the Immaculate Conception survived the burning of Atlanta.

During the 1864 siege this Irish immigrant attended soldiers of both armies and offered Mass on many occasions for Union Army Catholics. When Sherman planned to burn Atlanta, Father O'Reilly appealed to the federal authorities to spare his church. O'Reilly reportedly sent Sherman this threat: "If you burn the Catholic church, all Catholics in the ranks of the Union Army will mutiny."

He intervened to save City Hall and the Atlanta Courthouse as well. His efforts also saved four Protestant churches—Central Presbyterian, Trinity United Methodist, Second Baptist, and St. Philip's Episcopal. (Second Baptist and St. Philip's Episcopal have since moved farther out.)

1982, a fire gutted the building, which led to its rebuilding. Two priests rest in the crypt under the altar, including Father Thomas O'Reilly, who was the priest at the church during the war.

► Walk up the hill. On the right corner, you will see Central Presbyterian Church. Sherman's troops used the first building, completed in 1860, as a slaughterhouse during the occupation. The present building, in Early English Gothic Revival style, has stood since 1885.

► Turn right on Washington Street. You will pass the front of the State Capitol Building across the street.

Of Interest

A Unique Capitol

Atlanta became Georgia's fifth capital in 1867. The classical Renaissance–style State Capitol Building, completed in 1889, resembles the nation's Capitol. It is one of the few in the nation that has a cupola and a dome.

Georgians built their capitol out of Indiana limestone. You will see marble from North Georgia on the walls, floors, steps, and the cornerstone. The construction costs came in slightly under the $1-million budget; $118.43 remained in the treasury.

A colossal four-story portico, with stone pediment, supported by six Corinthian columns set on large stone piers, dominates the facade. The state seal, which depicts the phoenix, adorns the front of the building.

The building has a 237-foot dome, one of the most distinguished in the nation. A mule-drawn wagon train brought forty-three ounces of gold dust and nuggets down from Dahlonega, a town in North Georgia, to cover the dome in gold leaf. The dome was refurbished in 1981.

28

In 1977 the building became a National Historic Landmark. It has recently undergone a $63-million restoration project. More children walk through this building than visit all the state parks in Georgia combined.

The capitol has one of the best-tended lawns in town. During the bitter winter of 1962–63, when everything froze, the secretary of the state spent $600 on green dye to restore color to the brown grass.

►Turn right on Mitchell. Look straight down the hill on Washington to see the Trinity United Methodist Church, founded in 1861. Father O'Reilly helped spare the original building—then located at Washington and Mitchell Streets—during the Civil War. The church, a neo-Gothic structure built in 1912, is now in its third location. The elegant opaque stained-glass windows illustrate the Ten

Of Interest

Thar's Gold in Them Thar Hills!

Few persons know that the nation's first major gold rush took place in Georgia rather than in California. It happened in 1828 in Dahlonega, northeast of Atlanta. *Dahlonega* actually comes from the Cherokee word for "precious yellow metal." The well-known phrase "Thar's gold in them thar hills" came from that period as well. Men brought millions of dollars worth of the gold ore out of those mountains, often using primitive methods. Most of the men took off for California when prospectors found a richer gold seam there. Locals say that enough gold still remains to pave the square around the courthouse a foot deep.

Commandments, the stories of the Old and New Testaments, and the history of the church. The church claims that its 3,500-pipe organ is the finest in the South.

Trinity had the first "air conditioning" installed in a public building in Atlanta. Each Saturday an ice man brought several hundred pounds of ice and placed it in a pan in the bell tower. On Sunday morning, a fan was turned on to blow across the ice, thus cooling the air.

➤You will pass Atlanta City Hall, a fourteen-story tower building completed in 1930. General Sherman used the original house on this site as his headquarters during the time of the occupation. The building has a reinforced concrete skeleton that the architect covered with terracotta to distinguish it from the State Capitol Building. He got the idea for many of City Hall's lacy details from the Gothic cathedrals designed in Europe in the Middle Ages.

➤Cross Central.

➤Walk uphill and turn right on Pryor.

You are now at the Fulton County Government Center, an entire block defined by Peachtree, Mitchell, and Pryor Streets and Martin Luther King Jr. Drive. After the State Capitol Building on the right, you'll see the nine-story Fulton County Courthouse, the largest public structure built in the classical style in the city. The courthouse is also Georgia's largest. Completed in 1914, it is the county's third courthouse. The granite exterior covers a very modern, fireproof building.

➤Cross Martin Luther King Jr. Drive and Alabama Street. This will bring you to the Visitors Center and the end of the walk.

Walk 2

Five Points and Historic Downtown

   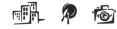

General location: In the heart of downtown near the entrance to Underground Atlanta.

Special attractions: Historic buildings, Woodruff Park.

Difficulty rating: Easy; mainly flat with one slight incline; all sidewalks.

Distance: 1 mile.

Estimated time: 30 minutes.

Services: Restaurants with rest rooms along the route for customers only; rest rooms in Atlanta–Fulton County Public Library and the Candler Building.

Restrictions: Dogs must be on leashes no longer than 6 feet, and their droppings must be picked up.

31

Five Points and Historic Downtown

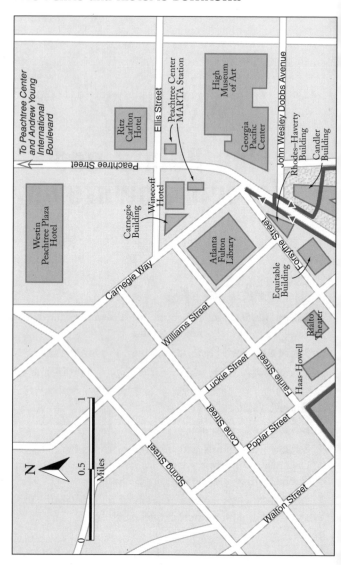

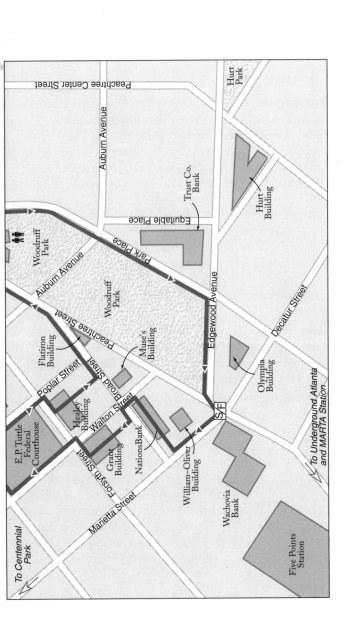

For more information: Call the Atlanta Convention and Visitors Bureau. The Atlanta Preservation Center conducts tours of this area March–November. Call for times and information.

Getting started: This walk starts at Five Points, the heart of downtown Atlanta. To reach Five Points from I–85/75 South, take exit 95, go to the second light and turn right onto Auburn. Take Auburn to Peachtree Street and turn left. Turn left onto Mitchell Avenue and left onto Central Avenue and park at Park 90 Central or at one of the two lots across the street. As you continue downhill, you may turn left on either Wall or Decatur Streets to find parking lots. Or you may turn left onto Washington Street off Mitchell and then turn left onto Martin Luther King Jr. Drive to two parking lots on that street.

From I–85/75 North take exit 94; then turn left at the second light onto Auburn Avenue. Follow directions above.

Public transportation: Take MARTA at the airport to the Five Points station. Turn left onto Peachtree Street after leaving the station and walk 0.2 mile to Five Points. Call MARTA for current schedules.

Overview: It is hard to picture downtown Atlanta as thick forest in a remote wilderness, but that is just what it looked like in its early days. Hardy Ivy, the first white settler, who came in 1833, bought a large plot of land for $225. In the forest that covered most of present downtown Atlanta, he built a cabin for his wife and five children.

After the state legislature approved the plan to establish a rail-line terminal point in 1836, the railroad came through the Five Points area. The small village grew from the Underground area to the Five Points area, where Marietta, Decatur, Peachtree, and Edgewood Streets converge.

The settlement resembled the Wild West, having more taverns than churches. Law and order barely existed.

By the latter half of the nineteenth century, the rich had built mansions there, called "Mansion Row." By 1900, however, commercial expansion and skyscrapers had pushed the home owners farther out.

On this walk you will trek Atlanta's highest point, Peachtree Ridge, at the confluence of three ridges. Rivers on the east of the ridge flow to the Atlantic, and those on the west flow to the Gulf of Mexico or the Mississippi River.

You will also notice odd-shaped lots, blocks, and buildings. These came about because streets followed old Indian trails, and railroad tracks also went at odd angles. You may also notice that only four streets meet at Five Points rather than five; at one time five Indian trails met there.

Now start walking on former Indian trails now filled with interesting buildings.

The Walk

➤Start at the corner of Peachtree and Marietta, where a plaque in the sidewalk reads: IN 1887 COCA COLA WAS FIRST SOLD AS A CARBONATED BEVERAGE FROM THE SODA FOUNTAIN AT JACOBSON'S DRUG STORE ACROSS THE STREET. The sculpture at the left, *Five Points*, by artist George Beasley, suggests the artesian well that at one time erupted here. The actual well was capped when the water was discovered, even back then, to be polluted.

➤Walk straight on Marietta. Across the street on the left you will see the Wachovia Bank tower. This black-steel high-rise sits on the ground where Jacob's Drugstore formerly stood.

➤ Pass the 1930 William-Oliver Building on the right. In the beautiful marble lobby with fine bronze work you'll find its original elevator. The barber shop has operated there since the building first opened.

Look up Marietta Street to see a statue of Henry Grady. Grady, editor of *The Atlanta Constitution*, helped rebuild the city after the Civil War.

➤ Enter the NationsBank Building—formerly the Empire Building—on the right. This building was the first in the city to be constructed with a steel frame. The banking hall remains as one of the greatest of its kind in the nation. Notice the giant Corinthian pilasters and the walls and floors that use eight kinds of marble. Gigantic chandeliers hang from the ceiling. Georgia State University's School of Business occupies the upper floors.

➤ Walk through the lobby and exit the building onto Walton Street.

➤ Turn left and cross Broad Street.

➤ Turn left and enter the Grant Building on the right. The 1898 building, one of the city's best examples of the Chicago style of commercial architecture, had a 1980 renovation.

➤ Walk through the lobby and exit the building.

➤ Turn right and cross Forsyth Street.

➤ Turn left and cross Walton Street.

➤ You will be facing the E. P. Tuttle Federal Courthouse and Post Office on the corner. This 1908 Stone Mountain granite building, designed in Second Renaissance Revival style, now houses the Eleventh Circuit Court of Appeals. E. P. Tuttle, one of the South's most famous judges, was instrumental in many civil rights issues around the region.

Walk 2

➤Walk straight on Walton Street to Fairlie Street. You are entering the 21-block Fairlie-Polar area, which has changed little since the early 1900s. It had its heyday around the turn of the twentieth century because of its location near the railroads.

➤Turn right on Fairlie and walk 1 short block to Poplar Street. View the Retail Credit Building diagonally across the street. This Art Deco–style building had the first air conditioning and underfloor wiring in the city.

➤Turn right on Poplar Street. View the Haas-Howell Building across the street. Neel Reid, popular Atlanta architect, designed the 1922 building to house the South's largest general insurance company. Bobby Jones, the famous amateur golfer, had his law office here.

At the corner look left to see the Rialto Theater. The original Rialto began as the Southeast's largest silent movie house in 1916, complete with the largest electric sign south of New York City. In the 1960s the movie facility was demolished and then rebuilt on the same site. Due to Atlanta's weakening downtown economy, the theater closed its doors in 1989. Georgia State University acquired it in the early 1990s and raised $14 million to restore it.

➤Cross Forsyth Street and turn right. Enter the Healey Building on the left. Developer William T. Healey had this elegant office tower built in 1913. The Tudor ornamentation and atrium lobby make it an outstanding example of the city's early skyscrapers. It used the Gothic style of the terra-cotta ornaments, the most fashionable for skyscraper design at that time. The building has its original light fixtures and its original barber shop.

➤Exit the building and turn left on Broad Street.

Of Interest

Trees Atlanta

As you walk, look for signs telling that "Trees Atlanta" planted certain trees. Since 1985 this nonprofit citizens' group has been improving and beautifying the urban environment by planting trees.

To get instant shade and visual impact, they plant large hardwood shade trees—22,000 since 1985—and evergreen magnolias and hollies. To handle pollution at its source (car exhaust), they have planted thousands of hardwood trees and evergreen magnolias along expressway corridors. Twenty large magnolias on I–75 at the Tenth Street Bridge create a gateway into the Georgia Institute of Technology.

The organization has also helped create several parks in the city. You may see one of them on this walk on International Boulevard by the Westin Peachtree Hotel.

More than 800 volunteers take part in the program, many giving their professional skills. Each fall and winter they plant thousands of trees in metro-area neighborhoods, at schools, and wherever trees are needed. They have also helped distribute 60,000+ saplings to area citizens to plant.

Trees Atlanta gives tree walks in various parts of the city. Call to see if one is scheduled during your visit.

➤Cross Poplar and Luckie Streets; then turn left on Peachtree Street. Look to the right across Broad to view the Flatiron Building at the corner of Broad and Peachtree Streets.

This eleven-story 1897 building at 74 Peachtree is Atlanta's oldest standing skyscraper. Its nickname comes from its narrow, triangular shape, which looks like a flat-iron from above.

On the left you will pass the Equitable Building. The columns in front of the building came from the original Equitable Life Assurance Company on Park Place. You will pass that site later on this walk.

➤Cross Williams Street.

➤Proceed uphill to the Rhodes-Haverty Building on the left and enter the lobby of the present Marriott Residence Inn. Amos G. Rhodes and James J. Haverty established an outstanding furniture company in 1873. They later had an amicable split, and the two companies still exist. This 1929 twenty-one-story building, Atlanta's tallest building until 1955, has a blend of Byzantine and Art Deco motifs. Take a look at the impressive Italian–style lobby ceiling, restored by one of the Fox Theater restorers.

➤Exit the building and turn left. You will pass the 1913 Hillyer Trust building at 140 Peachtree Street.

➤Continue walking uphill. You will pass Margaret Mitchell Square, a memorial to the author.

➤Look to the left to see the Atlanta–Fulton County Public Library, which occupies a full city block. It took more than ten years to complete, opening to the public in 1980. The library has a large *Gone With the Wind* collection.

➤Across Carnegie Way you will see the fourteen-story Winecoff Hotel, circa 1913. William Fleming Winecoff built one of the city's finest hotels, which, unfortunately, became famous for a fire—the worst in U.S. history—in 1946 that killed 119 people, including Winecoff. The victims died from smoke inhalation, and the fire led to changes in fire-safety regulations nationwide. Next door, the landmark 1927 Carnegie Building retains much of its original charm.

➤Look to the left on 141 Carnegie Way to see Scarlett Fever, a shop of *Gone With the Wind* goods. The shop has an eclectic assortment of *GWTW* movie memorabilia, gourmet foods (some canned especially for Scarlett Fever include Georgia Peach Spread), new and used books, and quilts. You'll find items such as Scarlett dolls—$40 and up—and, for a "Hotlanta" day, paper fans featuring the faces of Scarlett and Rhett. Just past a dollhouse replica of Tara, you will find the bookstore. Most books focus on Atlanta and Southern history.

➤Across Peachtree, you will see the fifty-two-story Georgia-Pacific Center. Built in 1982, it stands on the site of Loew's Grand Theater, the site of the world premiere of *Gone With the Wind*. You will find the downtown branch of the High Museum of Art located inside the Georgia-Pacific Center.

You are now close to three popular eating places. If you continue north on Peachtree Street for 1 block, you will find Planet Hollywood on the left corner of Andrew Young International Boulevard. If you turn left at that corner, you will find Pittypat's Porch, a longtime Southern-style restaurant. The cafeteria in the Georgia Pacific building serves employees primarily but also welcomes visitors.

➤Cross Peachtree Street at the crosswalk. Turn right and cross John Wesley Dobbs Avenue. Continue downhill on Peachtree Street and enter the Candler Building through an entryway on the left.

➤Exit the lobby through the Park Place Street entrance. Take a look at the fully clothed women over the portal.

The Candler Building

Mary Combs, the first black woman to own property in Atlanta, paid $250 for the site of this building. She sold it later for $500 to buy her husband's freedom. The Wesley Chapel, which later became the First Methodist Church in another location, formerly stood here.

Asa Candler erected this building in 1906, covering it in white marble, called "the white gold of Georgia." People considered Candler mad because he located the building so far from the city's commercial center. He also faced the building away from the railroad, another first. The neo-Renaissance building—the tallest (seventeen stories) and best-equipped office building in the city at that time—is considered one of Atlanta's most treasured architectural jewels and still has the original Tiffany windows.

Decorative sculpture on the exterior features street-level bays with medallions showing profiles of famous men. You will see barebreasted maidens over the portal on the Peachtree side, whereas those on the Park Place Street side wear clothing—Candler always took his mother through that entrance.

►Turn right and cross Auburn Avenue. You will be passing Woodruff Park on the right, a green space in the heart of the city. Robert W. Woodruff—head of Coca-Cola—gave much of his wealth to Atlanta, including land for this park. He preferred to remain anonymous, and Atlantans knew him as "Mr. Anonymous Donor."

The park features a 30-foot fountain, a waterfall, benches, and a music pavilion. Alcoholic beverages are prohibited.

Across Woodruff Park on Peachtree Street, view Muse's Building, identified by its rooftop neon sign that has beamed since 1939. George Muse came from New York in the 1880s and opened a clothing company, operating a store in this building from 1921 until 1992. A Confederate arsenal stood on that site during the Civil War.

You will pass the 1969 Trust Company Bank on the left. The Equitable Life Assurance Company, built in the 1890s, stood next door. That eight-story building was the first "skyscraper" in Atlanta. The three large columns that now stand in front of the bank came from the entrance to the old building.

➤When you reach the corner of Park Place and Edgewood Street, look left to see the Hurt Building, a prominent landmark on its elongated triangular site. Named after developer Joel Hurt, this seventeen-story, steel-frame building was finished in 1913. Marble Corinthian columns support the beautifully restored domed ceiling of the entrance rotunda. Remodeling enlarged the dramatic lobby, which showcases an ornate Violetta marble stairway and grillwork.

➤Turn right onto Edgewood Avenue. In the park you will see the bronze statue *From the Ashes*—the figure of a woman and a phoenix that represent Atlanta's comeback after the Civil War. The statue was moved from an obscure location to here for the Olympic Games in 1996.

➤Cross Peachtree Street and come to the end of the walk.

Look to the left to see Georgia State University, an urban research university, 2 blocks down Decatur Street. It is the second-largest institution in the university system of Georgia, currently enrolling more than 32,000 students annually. More than 1,000 students come from 117 foreign countries, and students come from forty-eight states. *U.S. News & World Report* named Georgia State's part-time M.B.A. program the fourth best in the nation.

In recent years Georgia State has been a leader in downtown revitalization. Its buildings replaced some of the city's worst slums: rows of pawnshops, cheap hotels, and rundown warehouses.

Of Interest

Other Walks

Peachtree Center

Continue north on Peachtree past the Winecoff Hotel to reach this impressive area from Ellis to Baker Streets. Architect John Portman, who changed Atlanta's landscape, built this Merchandise Mart complex in 1961. A skybridge connects office towers, hotels, and a shopping arcade.

The Hyatt Regency, with a twenty-story atrium in its lobby, caused a revolution in hotel design when it was built and brought Portman worldwide acclaim as an architect. The Marriott-Marquis Hotel and Towers has a forty-eight-story atrium in its lobby.

The Westin Peachtree Plaza—seventy-three stories and 723 feet tall—is the tallest hotel in the Western Hemisphere. You may take an elevator to the top and get a panoramic view of Atlanta and the outlying areas or eat in the revolving restaurant.

Peachtree Center MARTA station is located in a tunnel under the crest of Peachtree. The rough walls remain so that visitors can see how this engineering marvel was blasted from solid rock. One of the longest escalators in the country, 102 feet, leads from the station to Peachtree Street.

Centennial Olympic Park and CNN

Walk straight from Five Points on Marietta Street to Techwood Avenue to reach the twenty-one-acre park, which served as one of the most popular gathering spots during the 1996 Olympic Games. Since then, the Water Gardens and Quilt Plazas have joined the park's popular Fountain of Rings. Children would enjoy the run-through fountain.

The park—the largest center-city park developed in the nation since the mid-1970s—has become a permanent civic symbol and community focal point. The Fountain of Rings, which represents the Olympic symbol of five inter-connecting rings, is the world's largest fountain. A court displays twenty-four brilliantly colored flags: one Olympic flag and twenty-three flags that honor the host countries of the modern Olympic Games. Nearby stands the Centennial Tree, a one-hundred-year-old Georgia pecan tree that represents the 1996 Olympic celebration. The Bicentennial Tree stands nearby, symbolizing the next one hundred years of the Olympic Games.

The park also has a 1,200-seat amphitheater, a six-acre great lawn, and pathways of commemorative bricks that stitch together pieces of the park's landscape. The park opens daily, and concerts, children's events, and other activities take place there.

CNN, home of Ted Turner's broadcasting empire, lies across the street and conducts free tours daily.

Walk 3

Sweet Auburn/ Martin Luther King Jr. Historic Site and Preservation District

General location: The walk starts about 1 1/4 miles east of downtown.

Special attractions: The Martin Luther King Jr. Historic Site, historic churches and buildings, a library, and a museum.

Difficulty rating: Easy; mainly level with one moderate hill; all on sidewalks.

45

Sweet Auburn/Martin Luther King Jr. Historic Site and Preservation District

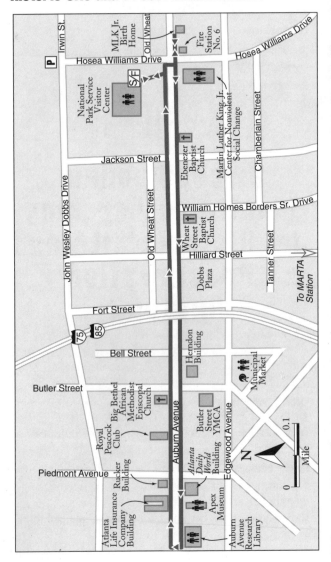

Walk 3

Distance: 2.3 miles.

Estimated time: 1 hour, 10 minutes.

Services: Rest rooms at tourist information center; restaurants on Auburn Avenue.

Restrictions: Dogs must be on leashes 6 feet or less in length, and their droppings must be picked up. The park is open every day from 9:00 A.M. to 5:00 P.M.; closed New Year's Day and Christmas. In January and periods of heavy visitation, the park may extend hours.

For more information: Call the Atlanta Convention and Visitors Bureau and the National Park Service Visitor Center.

Getting started: This walk begins at the National Park Service Visitor Center, 450 Auburn Avenue. To reach the center from I–85/75 South, take exit 248C. At the end of the exit ramp, go straight to the second light. Turn left onto Auburn. Follow signs 0.6 mile to the site. From I–85/75 North, take exit 94. At the end of the exit ramp, go straight ahead of the second traffic light. Turn right onto Auburn and follow signs 0.5 mile to the site. Turn left at Hosea Williams Drive and follow the signs for ample visitors' parking. In some sections of Auburn, free parking is available along the street, and you will find some off-street parking throughout the neighborhood.

Public transportation: Take MARTA bus route 3 east from the Five Points station to the King Memorial station; then walk or take the bus the half-mile to the site. Call MARTA for current schedules and confirm a bus's destination when you buy the ticket.

Overview: Hardy Ivy was the first white man to own property in Atlanta. He bought property that included an Indian trail that became Auburn Avenue in 1893.

German-Americans owned most of the area businesses and residences at that time, and their servants and slaves lived there, too.

After the Civil War Atlanta experienced general integration. Nearly half a century later, however, different factors led to the neighborhoods separating by race. A 1906 race riot led to blacks withdrawing into their own neighborhoods. Black businesses on Peachtree dwindled even as they flourished on Auburn. The 1917 Atlanta fire cleared most of the land between Edgewood and Ponce de Leon. The vacant land left by the fire allowed Auburn Avenue to become the commercial center of the growing African-American neighborhood there.

Auburn went by the name "the Black Peachtree Street." John Wesley Dobbs, considered "mayor" of Auburn Avenue, coined the phrase "Sweet Auburn" in the 1930s. Auburn had the most African-American financial institutions of any street in America. In 1956 *Fortune* magazine reported that Auburn Avenue "is the richest Negro street in the world."

Sweet Auburn helped produce its most famous son, Martin Luther King Jr., leader of the civil rights movement. In 1980 Congress created the twenty-three-acre King historic site to memorialize King and his ideals of justice, equality, and freedom. The National Park Service has designated a portion of this district as a National Historic Site. The district retains much of its residential and architectural character of the period 1929–1941, when King lived there.

Now get walking. A rich experience awaits you.

The Walk

➤Start at the National Park Service Visitor Center and pick up a map for the district. The center shows two videos about King's life and one just for children. A walk-through exhibit, "The Courage of Leadership: The Life of Martin Luther King Jr.," has sections with photographs and a TV monitor above each showing film footage of a civil rights march. A gift shop offers books, tapes, and posters for sale.

➤As you leave the Visitor Center, turn right and walk uphill to Auburn. On the plaza in front of the building, you will see a statue entitled *Behold*. Sculptor Patrick Morelli drew inspiration from the ancient African ritual of a father lifting a newborn child to heaven while reciting the words, "Behold the only thing greater than yourself."

➤Turn left onto Auburn and walk uphill.

➤Turn right and cross Auburn.

➤Cross Hosea Williams Drive. At the corner stands Fire Station Number Six, one of Atlanta's oldest fire stations. Register inside for free Martin Luther King Jr. Birth Home tours.

Next door to the fire station stands Our Lady of Lourdes Catholic Church—organized in 1912—which conducted one of the city's few schools for black children. Supposedly the nuns chased Martin Luther King Jr. and his childhood friends away from the playground.

➤Walk uphill to the Birth Home, 501 Auburn. King's maternal grandfather, the Reverend Alfred Williams, bought this 1895 home in 1909. The King family lived here until 1941, and King was born here on January 15, 1929. The house has many of the original furnishings.

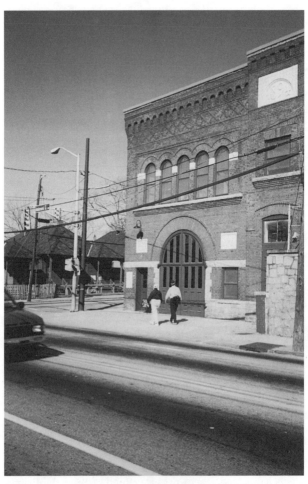

Visitors may register for free tours of the Martin Luther King Jr. Birth Home at Fire Station Number 6, one of the oldest fire stations in Atlanta.

Across the street you will see some restored circa 1905 "shotgun" houses. Shotgun houses got their names from the fact that anyone who stood at the front door could look straight through to the back door. Many low-income families lived in this type of housing in Southern cities around 1900.

Of Interest

Auburn's Most Famous Son

Martin Luther King Jr. grew up in a family that valued education. He loved books and words even before he learned to read. Supposedly, instead of settling disputes with friends with fists, he would say, "I'm going to get me some big words."

King graduated from Morehouse College in Atlanta at age nineteen. He later received a bachelor of divinity degree from Crozer Theological Seminary and a Ph.D. in theology from Boston University. In Boston he met Coretta Scott and married her in June 1953.

Dr. King later went to Montgomery, Alabama, to serve as a pastor. He became the leader of the Montgomery Improvement Association after blacks boycotted the buses there.

Having admired Mahatma Gandhi's philosophy of nonviolent resistance, Dr. King visited India in 1957 to study those teachings firsthand. In 1960 he moved to Atlanta and became president of the new Southern Christian Leadership Conference. In 1963 he led a march on Washington, D.C., where he delivered his famous "I Have a Dream" speech.

In 1964 he received the Nobel Peace Prize for his tireless work for civil rights. In April 1968 he went to Memphis to take part in a sanitation workers' strike. An assassin fatally shot him on April 4.

Keeping the Dream Alive

As you walk down the steps off Auburn, you enter the King Center courtyard. The architecture recalls Mahatma Ghandi's influence on Dr. King's life.

King's widow, Coretta Scott King, and his sister Christine King Farris started the center in Mrs. King's basement in 1968. After King's assassination the women wanted a "living memorial" dedicated to preserving his legacy. The center, which opened in 1982, houses the most extensive collection of King memorabilia in the world.

Freedom Hall contains the gift shop and the museum. The museum contains a small display of King's clothing and personal items, including his Nobel Prize medal. You will even see the perfectly preserved cuff-link collection of this man who always dressed with care. A photographic chronology of his life, including pictures of him as a toddler, lines the walls.

The Freedom Walkway runs parallel to the pool. You will walk through a progressive visual sequence of architectural spaces that gradually leads to a meditative space focused on Dr. King's tomb. The simple white Georgia-marble crypt sits within a circular brick platform at the center of a narrow pool. The bright blue pool, reflecting the heavens and the gravesite, symbolizes the River of Life. The inscription on the crypt carries a variation of a phrase from his "I Have a Dream" speech, delivered on the steps of the Lincoln Memorial. Those words read: FREE AT LAST! FREE AT LAST! THANK GOD ALMIGHTY, I'M FREE AT LAST!

On the left you pass the Chapel of All Faiths. On the far side of the pool, a brick cylinder hosting the eternal flame stands directly in front of the crypt. Next to the flame is a tree that Dr. King supposedly played on as a child.

Walk 3

➤As you leave the house, turn left and walk downhill on Auburn.

➤Cross Hosea Williams Drive.

➤You will pass the Martin Luther King Jr. Center for Nonviolent Social Change.

Of Interest

Historic Ebenezer Baptist Church

A. D. Williams, Dr. King's maternal grandfather, became the second pastor of this church in 1894. He remained pastor until his death in 1931.

In segregated Atlanta, Williams took an active role in advancing rights for blacks. The Atlanta Branch of the NAACP (National Association for the Advancement of Colored People) met first at Ebenezer. Williams served as president of that organization.

Martin Luther King Sr. married Alberta, one of the Reverend Williams's daughters. Called "Daddy King" by the church members, he took over as pastor after Williams's death. A fiery personality, he fought against segregation.

Ebenezer gave birth to the Southern Christian Leadership Conference, an organization of churches and religious leaders. Martin Luther King Jr. became its first president.

King went to Sunday school at Ebenezer as a child and received his ordination there in 1947. From 1960 until his death, he shared pastoral duties with his father. His funeral took place there on April 10, 1968.

An assassin shot Alberta King to death one Sunday in 1974.

Martin Luther King Jr.'s widow, Coretta Scott King, and his sister still attend the church.

➤You will pass Ebenezer Baptist Church at 407 Auburn. You may enter the Educational Building to take tours of the church or to purchase items from the souvenir shop. You may hear interpretative talks on church history, sermons and speeches of Dr. King and his father, and choral music. The church does not charge for visits but appreciates donations. Look across the street to see the new $8-million building Ebenezer now occupies.

➤Cross Jackson. You are now leaving the Martin Luther King Jr. Historic District.

➤Cross William Holmes Borders Sr. Drive. The 1881 Wheat Street Baptist Church sits on the corner. In 1957 police arrested Reverend William Holmes Borders, pastor, as well as six other ministers, in their "Leadership" movement. Their actions led to the desegregation of Atlanta's public transportation system.

➤Cross Hilliard Street.

➤You will pass Dobbs Plaza on the left, named for John Wesley Dobbs. People called Dobbs, born in 1882, the "mayor" of Auburn Avenue. Proud of Atlanta blacks' business success, he coined the phrase "sweet Auburn." At the time of his death, he was one of Georgia's best-known black leaders. His grandson, Maynard Jackson, became Atlanta's first black mayor in 1974.

The plaza's design symbolically links elements of African history with the history of blacks as reflected in Dobbs's achievements and the community.

➤Cross Fort Street. You will walk under I–85/75.

➤Cross Bell Street.

➤At the corner you will pass the mini-police precinct at 247 Auburn. The city hired its first black policemen in

1948, eighty years after the black community first asked for them.

➤You will pass the Herndon Building at 239 Auburn. Alonzo F. Herndon erected this building in 1926 for his Atlanta Life Insurance Company.

Of Interest

Alonzo F. Herndon

Herndon, born in 1858—son of a slave and her master—spent his first seven years as a slave in Georgia. He could have passed for white because of his fair skin. After emancipation he went to work in a barbershop to help feed his family. He later owned barbershops in Atlanta, the largest—called a "tonsorial palace"—located on Peachtree Street. Called the most glamorous in the world, that shop incorporated ideas he learned while visiting barbershops in some European countries. It had marble floors, chandeliers, and two walls lined with mirrors. The place catered to whites only.

Herndon branched out into real estate and then bought a small insurance association in 1905. By the time of his death in 1927, he had become Atlanta's first black millionaire and one of the South's wealthiest blacks. A philanthropist, Herndon supported, often anonymously, many Atlanta causes.

Herndon's wife, Adrienne, performed Shakespeare for black audiences and taught elocution at Atlanta University. Herndon built a mansion near the campus, where he commissioned a series of murals enshrining his up-from-slavery saga on the living-room walls. One of them shows a boy standing with his mother in front of a log cabin. You may visit the 1910 Herndon Beaux Arts–style home on Walk 13.

➤When you reach Butler Street, look left to see the Municipal Market of Atlanta, which opened in 1924. At that time segregation laws did not allow blacks to shop inside, so owners set up stalls outside to sell to blacks. The market has several eateries.

On the right you will see the Butler Street YMCA, which started in 1864 in the basement of Wheat Street Baptist Church. It is the only minority YMCA in America that has never been a branch of another. The Hungry Club Forum formed secretly there in 1948 to bring blacks and whites together to discuss business and social cases. Race laws at the time prohibited the two races from eating together in public. Those meetings helped ease Atlanta's desegregation. The group later met openly.

➤Cross Butler. This area of Auburn Avenue had the largest concentration of black financial institutions in America in the 1930s.

Poro Beauty School, 177 Auburn, was once part of the leading chain of black beauty schools in the nation.

You will pass the office of *The Atlanta Daily World*, at 145 Auburn. William Alexander Scott, II, started the paper in 1928. In 1932 it became the first black *daily* published in the United States, and it is the longest-running such paper. Scott ran newspapers during a time when blacks didn't get into mainstream newspapers. He used the paper to crusade against the Ku Klux Klan, Georgia's poll tax and white primary, and Atlanta's segregated Police Department. Family members still run it.

You will then pass the APEX (African American Panoramic Experience), Atlanta's only African-American museum. It houses a collection of African and black arts.

You will then reach the Auburn Avenue Research Library of Black Culture & History.

➤Cross the street and make a return trip up Auburn to the Visitor Center. At 148 Auburn you will pass the Atlanta Life Insurance Company Building that Alonzo Herndon started. From 1920 to 1980 this served as the headquarters of the country's largest black-owned stockholder life insurance company.

On the corner you will pass the Rucker Building, the first that blacks financed and built in Atlanta. On the wall you will see a photographic display of Atlanta leaders.

➤Cross Piedmont. Look left to see Citizens Trust Bank, which Heman Perry launched. People called Perry—who grew up in poverty and later became a financial genius—the "black Booker T. Washington."

➤The park at the corner of Piedmont Avenue was named for John Calhoun, a successful black businessman.

You will pass the Royal Peacock Club, which opened in 1930. It catered primarily to blacks, who couldn't attend white-owned clubs.

At 198–202 Auburn, you will pass Cornelius King Realty Company. It started as one of Heman Perry's ventures and has operated on Auburn Avenue more than seventy years. The 1915 Silver Moon Barber Shop in this building bears the words OLDEST BLACK SHOP IN ATLANTA.

At the corner of Auburn and Butler, you will pass the 1868 Big Bethel African Methodist Episcopal, A.M.E., Church. The blue JESUS SAVES sign shines from the church's steeple, Sweet Auburn's most visible landmark. Slave owners founded this—the first black church in Atlanta—in 1847. The church housed the first school for black children in Atlanta in its basement in 1879. Morris Brown College started here in 1881, the only college blacks founded in Georgia. You can visit the campus on Walk 13.

➤You will pass the 1912 Odd Fellows Building, Auditorium, and Tower, built by the wealthiest black fraternal order in Atlanta.

At 328 Auburn you will find the 1927 Tabor Building, a fine example of African-American handicraft and artisan work with ornamental Italian tile facings. At present the building houses the Women's Division of the Southern Christian Leadership Conference.

The next building of interest is the 1937 Prince Hall Masonic Building. The Southern Christian Leadership Conference, organized in the 1950s, still operates from this building. WERD, the nation's first black-owned and licensed radio station, also broadcasts from this building.

You will pass two funeral homes, both founded by black women. The Jim Crow laws extended to the cemeteries and funeral homes, so blacks had to start their own.

➤Continue until you reach the Visitor Center and the end of the walk.

Walk 4

Historic Oakland Cemetery

   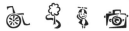

General location: This cemetery lies 1 mile east of downtown.

Special attractions: One of the finest Victorian cemeteries in the United States with curved drives and walkways shaded by ancient trees that give it parklike qualities. Visitors with limited time may want to visit Margaret Mitchell's grave only. From the entrance gate take the first left street. Turn left at the first driveway; then turn right at the sign pointing to the grave.

Difficulty rating: Mostly level, with some inclines.

Distance: 1.5 miles.

Estimated time: 45 minutes.

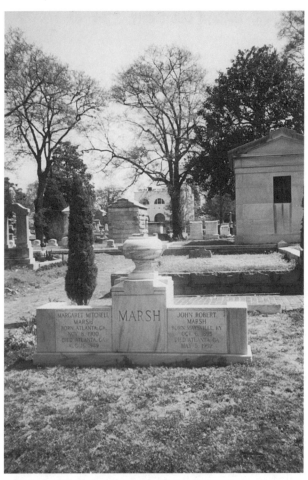

The grave of author Margaret Mitchell draws the most visitors to Historic Oakland Cemetery. She is buried with her husband, John Robert Marsh.

Historic Oakland Cemetery

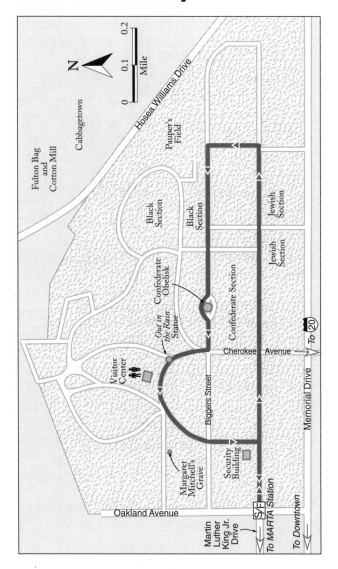

Services: You may bring a picnic to the cemetery, or hike or jog there. The Visitors' Center in the Bell Tower Building has rest rooms and free brochures. At the center you may purchase maps with information on more than fifty cemetery sites. Historic Oakland Cemetery, Inc., conducts guided tours regularly for a fee. Groups get special rates. You will find welcome water fountains throughout the cemetery.

Restrictions: Do not park on the grass or walkways. Avoid those areas where funerals are taking place. Take photographs or make sketches, but make no stone rubbings. Walk only on the walkways. Do not sit, stand, or walk on walls or monuments. One adult must accompany every twenty children over the age of ten and every ten children under the age of ten. Dogs must be on leashes no longer than 6 feet, and their droppings must be picked up.

For more information: Call Historic Oakland Cemetery.

Getting started: Take I–75/85, exit 248A south to Martin Luther King Jr. Drive, or take I–20 from downtown east to Hosea Williams Drive exit 59A; then drive north to Memorial Drive. Look for the entrance on Oakland Avenue on the right. You may park in the cemetery only on the asphalt-paved driveways near the Visitors' Center. Buses may park on Oakland Avenue.

Public transportation: Take an eastbound MARTA train to the King Memorial station. Exit the station onto DeKalb Avenue; then turn left onto Grant Street. Walk 0.2 mile; then turn left onto Martin Luther King Jr. Drive, which dead-ends at the cemetery gates after 0.1 mile. Call MARTA for current schedules and confirm the bus/train destination when you buy the ticket.

Overview: Oakland Cemetery, founded in 1850, is Atlanta's oldest municipal cemetery and its richest historic site. It originally covered six acres, and it now has expanded to eighty-eight. Since the city had no public parks at the time of Oakland's founding, Oakland became a "park," where residents picnicked on Sunday afternoons.

Between 1850 and 1884 nearly all burials—about 100,000—took place here. Slaves, soldiers, farmers, businessmen, paupers, millionaires, the unknown, and the famous rest here. Nearly 3,000 soldiers, many unknown, lie here. Oakland has white, black, and Jewish sections, as well as a paupers' field. The large numbers of children's graves tell of the high infant mortality rate of the mid-nineteenth century.

During the Civil War the Union Army vandalized the cemetery. After the war the city council rebuilt the cemetery. During the eighteenth century, people buried their dead close together and neglected the cemetery. During the nineteenth century, however, a "rural cemetery movement" took place, which started in Boston. People placed graves with open space between them. The peacefulness of cemeteries also spoke of the Christian promise of eternal life.

The cemetery has unusual epitaphs, ornate Victorian statuary, and stained glass in the sixty elaborate mausoleums. The statues make the cemetery look like an outdoor art museum. As the Victorians became wealthy, they built big homes and big cemetery monuments. They also used many symbols on their graves. Much of the memorial art at Oakland, such as angels, points to a belief in victory over death. Victorian Atlantans combined pagan symbolism and classical symbolism along with their Christian beliefs in the visual images on tombstones.

Look for these symbols as you walk. The rose meant love; the lily-of-the-valley meant innocence; the acanthus leaf meant garden of heaven; and the palm leaf spoke of new life. A weeping willow symbolized sorrow; and a willow with a broken branch meant a life shortened by an early death, as did the rosebud. The urn represented the Greek symbol of mourning; drapery represented grief. A seashell spoke of rebirth. The dove symbolized the messenger of God carrying the soul to heaven.

By the late 1800s, the cemetery had no more space, and Atlanta established other cemeteries. Burials still take place in Oakland in spaces that families bought years ago.

Since 1976 Oakland Cemetery has been on the National Register of Historic Places. The 1896 wall has undergone an authentic restoration. Volunteer gardeners care for graves and use historically correct plantings.

Now start walking. You will enjoy stepping back in time into Victorian Atlanta.

The Walk

➤Start at the 1896 red brick entrance gate.

On the left you will see "cradle graves" that resemble beds. These emphasized the belief that the dead were only sleeping.

On the right you will see the grave of Sarah Todd Ivy. Her husband, Hardy Ivy, was the first white person to buy land in what is now downtown Atlanta. Hardy Ivy died in 1842, and therefore is buried elsewhere. You may read about Ivy in Walk 2.

Next on the right you see the grave of Martha Lumpkin. Before Atlanta had its present name, it went by Marthasville, named after Martha.

➤Continue along the main drive. Look downhill on the right to see the mausoleum with the Arch monument designed in Egyptian Revival–style architecture, which had become popular during that time.

When you reach the cross drive, you have reached the end of the original six acres, which go to the wall on the right and to the next drive on the left. Houses filled the surrounding area during the Civil War.

Look to the right—then into the last walkway on the left—to see the graves of Bobby Jones and his wife against the wall. Jones was perhaps the greatest amateur golfer in history.

➤Continue straight. You will be passing the Confederate section on the left. Here lie 2,500 Confederate and twenty Union soldiers, even though tradition forbade burying enemies side by side. During that hot 1864 August, however, Southerners could not locate the families of the enemy dead, so they buried them here. CSA on the marker refers to the Confederate States Army.

On the right you will pass the first Jewish section, where the city donated six plots in 1878. This is the second-oldest Jewish burial ground in Georgia, preceded only by Savannah's Jewish cemetery. Look for Hebrew inscriptions and symbols on the headstones. Raised hands identify the deceased as a *Kohen*, a descendant of Aaron and the high priests who officiated in the ancient temple. The pitcher and basin mark the grave of a *Levi*, a descendant of the Biblical tribe that assisted the high priests as temple functionaries. The Star of David became popular with the advent of the Zionist movement in the late nineteenth century. Russian Jews used this symbol at Oakland more than any others did. Many Jews took an active part in Masonic orders, so you will see Masonic symbols on some graves. Nearer the wall, you will see the 1892 Temple addition of the Jewish section, noticeable for the closely spaced graves. The poorer Russian Jews placed their graves closely together.

Past that section you will find the 1878 addition on the right that has ten lots. The German-Jewish community desired to fit into the culture of Victorian America and used elaborate landscaping, statuary art, and mausoleums.

➤At the top of the hill, turn left onto the driveway. On the right you will see the Inman plot. The husband/father was an ancestor of the man for whom Inman Park was named. You may read about that in Walk 9. Notice Little Hugh and Louise; these angels' faces show actual portraits of the children.

➤Walk downhill and turn left at the street. You will pass Paupers' Field on the right. Since the field has few markers, people thought it was empty. A researcher, however, found 17,000 graves.

Behind the field you will see the Fulton Bag and Cotton Mill.

Of Interest

Fulton Bag and Cotton Mill

The Fulton Bag and Cotton Mill operated from 1881 until 1977. The scene in *Gone With the Wind* that showed the blowing up of a munitions factory took place there.

As rural employment dried up in the early twentieth century, the mill attracted workers from Appalachia and rural Georgia. The mill provided adults and children tough, steady work for decades, producing cotton sacks for agricultural feed and other products. The people created a tight-knit community of 2,000, who lived in a cluster of "shotgun" houses that sprang up around the mill. Shotgun houses get their name from the fact that a person could stand in the front door and shoot a gun and the bullet would go straight through the house and out the back door.

Outsiders started calling the village Cabbagetown, possibly because of the continual smell of cooking cabbage. The people stayed to themselves and retained their Appalachian speech patterns and customs.

When the mill closed, it sent Cabbagetown and its generations of families into economic depression. Time and weather reduced the mill's eleven buildings to deteriorating hulks, and the neighborhood developed a reputation for crime and drugs.

In 1998 a $45-million redevelopment of eight mill buildings into loft apartments opened. On completion this will be one of the largest residential historic restoration projects in the nation.

Cabbagetown is listed on the National Register of Historic Places.

►You are passing the black section on the right. Carrie Steel Logan lies beneath the round monument. After the Civil War Logan worked at a railroad station, where she saw abandoned black children. She cared for them during the day and started taking some home at night. In 1888 she started the first black orphanage in the United States. She sold her house and did everything possible to raise money. The Carrie Steel–Pitts Home still exists.

Anton Graves, who became wealthy in real estate, rests in the only mausoleum in the black section.

The rust-colored headstone belongs to Bishop Wesley Gaines of the African Methodist Episcopal Church. Gaines assisted in the founding of Morris Brown College.

►Continue walking uphill. You will pass the *Lion of the Confederacy* on the right, a memorial to the approximately

2,500 unknown dead. The Atlanta Ladies Memorial Association commissioned the sculpture of the lion, a symbol of courage. T. M. Brady sculpted the fifteen-ton lion from a single piece of North Georgia marble.

➤Continue walking uphill. You will come to the monument in honor of "Our Confederate Dead." The Atlanta Ladies Memorial Association dedicated the Stone Mountain granite obelisk on April 26, 1874. The Romanesque-style shaft, unveiled four years later, stands 65 feet tall, at the time taller than any other Atlanta structure.

➤Bear right and continue uphill. Look up to the top of the hill to see the most imposing mausoleum in the cemetery at its highest point. The Gothic Revival structure, made of Italian marble, cost $80,000 in the 1890s. It would cost $300,000 now.

➤Turn right at the first drive. Look for the Boyd plot in the triangle straight ahead. On the lower side find the grave of Georgia Harris. This is one of two documented cases of black interments in the white sections of the cemetery. The Boyds had such strong feelings of affection for their domestic worker that they received permission for her burial.

➤Continue uphill to see the statue *Out in the Rain,* which allows rain to sprinkle over an umbrella covering two children. This statue copies an original shown in the 1876 Philadelphia centennial celebration. Because it had some minor damage, it cost only $96.80. A 1984 restoration cost $5,000.

On the left you will see the grave of Moses W. Formwalt, the first mayor of Atlanta. He also functioned as DeKalb County's sheriff; unfortunately, a prisoner stabbed him to death during a transporting.

➤Bear left and walk downhill past the Visitor Center, which has a museum and souvenir shop in the 1899 Bell Tower building. The cemetery stored bodies in the cellar until the time of their funerals. Iron bars kept out thieves who wanted to steal jewelry.

You will pass the Gray marker. The weeping woman recalls the myth of Niobe, whom the gods turned to stone as she wept for her slain children.

Look to the right at the first street to see the Romanesque-style mausoleum that looks most like a cathedral of any other here. It has a beautiful stained-glass window in its apse.

➤Bear left at the curve past the first driveway. Follow the signs to Margaret Mitchell's grave in the plot of the Marsh family, her husband's family. Her burial took place on August 17, 1949, a hot, humid day. Crowds swarmed outside while the 300 invited guests attended the funeral, but they rushed inside afterward, snatching funeral flowers as souvenirs.

➤Retrace your steps and turn right at the street. Walk uphill to the main street and turn right to go to the gate. This ends the walk.

Of Interest

Take Time to View the Roses

At the time of Oakland's founding, flowering beds of snapdragons, foxgloves, dusty millers, pansies, and roses covered its ground. A canopy of water oaks, maples, and magnolias shaded brick lanes. Family members developed elaborate gardens on the plots and came out regularly to tend them. By 1994, however, people had forgotten Oakland. The cemetery had few plants; its walls, sidewalks, and grave markers crumbled. Different professionals and volunteers came to the rescue, taking part in the Adopt-a-Plot program to preserve and beautify graveyards. They clear out weeds, dig, haul in soil, plant flowers, and do research to plant native and heirloom plants.

During February and March, you may see daffodils, which symbolize "regards." Some have been there for one hundred years; some are new.

When you visit Bobby Jones's grave, look for lilies that match the flowers engraved on his headstone. Notice the eighteen trees and other plants that form a horseshoe around the grave. A miniature circle of grass looks a little like a hole on a golf course. Pink fairy roses—a flower that was introduced in the 1930s as Jones's career was peaking—surround the green.

At the Confederate Obelisk look for the banana trees, elephant's ears, caladiums, cannas, and coleuses, all brightly colored exotics popular at the turn of the century.

When you reach the fountain, look across to the left to see the Butterfly Garden. Every plant provides nourishment for either the caterpillar or the butterfly. The butterfly is the symbol of the soul, resurrection, and rebirth.

The Margaret Mitchell plot features the fairy rose, a light-pink rose that was common in 1932, when she wrote *Gone With the Wind*. It blooms March–November. The perennial border is planted with the 'Whirling Butterflies' variety of gaura. Commonly known as wandflower, it blooms in the summer.

Walk 5

Grant Park: Zoo Atlanta

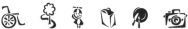

General location: About 2 miles southeast of downtown.

Special attractions: The zoo features 250 species of animals living in natural habitats—primarily from Africa and Southeast Asia, whose climates match Atlanta's.

Difficulty rating: Easy; some inclines; all on sidewalks.

Distance: 0.8 mile.

Estimated time: 30 minutes.

Services: Food and snacks are available at several venues, and rest rooms are located within the zoo. The zoo provides wheelchairs for its handicapped facilities. A gift shop has unique gifts, souvenirs, and necessities.

Grant Park: Zoo Atlanta

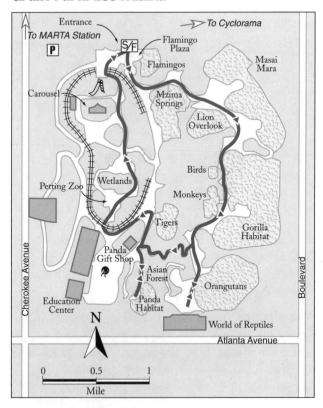

Restrictions: No dogs allowed. Tickets to see the pandas have a specific time for viewing.

For more information: Call Zoo Atlanta. Pick up a map when you purchase your ticket.

Getting started: From downtown take I–20 East to exit 59A. Turn south onto Hosea Williams Drive. Travel 0.3 mile;

then turn right at the second light onto Atlanta Avenue. After 0.1 mile turn right on Cherokee Avenue. Turn right into parking lots.

Public transportation: Take MARTA bus route 31 Grant Park/Lindbergh from Five Points, Peachtree Center, and Lindbergh rapid-rail stations. The King Memorial rapid-rail station is located near Oakland Cemetery, about ³/₄ mile north of Grant Park. After exiting the station turn left onto Grant Street.

Call MARTA for current schedules, and confirm the bus/train's destination when you buy the ticket.

Overview: Zoo Atlanta is one of the oldest continually operating zoos in the country. The zoo opened in 1889 when a traveling circus broke down in Atlanta. A local man, G. V. Gress, bought the animals and gave them to the city. Those animals included an African lion, California pumas, wildcats, monkeys, Backtrian and Dromedary camels, and a black bear. The zoo later added raccoons, hyenas, jaguars, elk, and gazelles.

The zoo went through a difficult period during the 1980s. In 1984 the Humane Society of the United States conducted a survey and named the zoo one of the ten worst zoos in the nation. A great deal of publicity followed this report, which led to the zoo's transformation into its present status as a world-class facility. In 1998 *Good Housekeeping* magazine named it as one of the top ten zoos in the nation.

The zoo layout consists of two attached circles, somewhat resembling the shape of a butterfly, with the main, upper-left wing larger than the other. You will find the smaller one downhill on the right.

Animals may not always be visible when you walk through the zoo. In general, animals come out first thing in the morning and late in the afternoon. They often rest during the middle of the day. The animals' activities vary according to different weather conditions and during different seasons. Scheduled feeding times provide an excellent opportunity to see the gorillas, at 1:30 P.M., and the orangutans, at 2:30 and 2:45 P.M. Elephant performances take place daily at 11:00 A.M. and 2:00 P.M. Try to visit the exhibit again if you should miss seeing the animals.

School groups come especially on Friday, and families come on Saturdays and Sundays. Come earlier in the week if you want to visit the zoo at a less-crowded time.

Now get walking. You will use all your senses to enjoy the animals of varied sizes, shapes, and colors that live here.

The Walk

►The walk starts at the Plaza, which you enter after you purchase your ticket. On the left you will see Flamingo Plaza. Approximately sixty Chilean flamingos stay here at all times. A male wears a leg band with an identifying number on his left leg; a female wears one on the right leg. Zookeepers supplement the flamingos' food with beta-carotene to preserve their pink color.

►Walk uphill and turn left. You may cross the bridge to enter Mzima Springs. The area names come from the animals' homes in Africa. You first see African elephants. Visitors express surprise at seeing red elephants instead of gray ones; the animals turn red from rolling in the Georgia clay. Three female "teenage" elephants live in a naturalistic habitat designed to mimic their African watering hole, Mzima Springs.

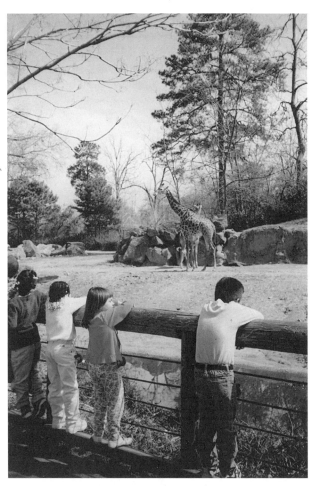

Children enjoy watching the giraffes at Zoo Atlanta.

Starlet O'Hara—born at the zoo and one of three female African elephants there—has outstanding painting abilities. Starlet began her painting career in 1989 with the help of a Georgia Tech graduate student who was researching elephant intelligence. Her colorful, broad-stroked watercolors have commanded prices as high as $1,800 at charity auctions. The zoo's elephant keepers now help Starlet with her paintings, which sell for about $15 to $25.

Farther on you might glimpse black rhinos, ostriches, gazelles, giraffes, zebras, cranes, and lions.

Zulu, a male lion born in 1991, is the "pride" of Zoo Atlanta. His roar can be heard up to 5 miles away. In the wild lions live in prides, sharing food usually caught by the females. Also in the wild many lions die as cubs, and adults often perish by age ten from attacks by people, other lions, or prey animals. In zoos they can live to twenty-five years or more. In captivity lions sometimes mate with tigers! A male lion and a female tiger produce a "liger." A female lion and a male tiger produce a "tigon."

As you continue straight, you will reach the Ford African Rain Forest, habitat of the gorillas. Moats separate the four gorilla habitats. Each group has one silverback (male), one female, and young gorillas. Early each morning, keepers scatter fruit so that the gorillas must forage as they would in the wild.

➤On the right is the exotic birds section. You may go into the building or stay on the path and come to the Sanaga Overlook on the right. You can watch the birds and the monkeys of Makokou. The drills—small African monkeys—are the most endangered primates in Africa. The only breeding pair in the United States lives here.

➤On the left you can look into the gorillas' habitat from a different side.

Willie B.'s Offspring

In the Ford African Rain Forest, you will see the statue of the famous gorilla Willie B., who came to the zoo in the spring of 1961. Then three years old, an animal dealer had caught him in the wilds of Africa's Congo. He died in February 2000.

In the spring of 1988, the Ford African Rain Forest opened. This habitat simulates the rain forests of the gorilla's native Africa, with the animals living in natural social groups.

After twenty-seven years of solitary existence, Willie B. moved into the forest. He socialized so successfully with female gorillas that he became the oldest-known reproducing male gorilla in captivity. He tied for second place as the oldest male western lowland gorilla in captivity in North America.

Willie B. fathered four offspring, and each had a different mother. All these gorillas have become quite famous. Female Kudzoo arrived in February 1994. What made her birth so significant? Both her parents originated from the wild population in Africa, making them "founder" animals. Since Choomba, the mother, had only one other offspring and Willie B. had none, Kudzoo brought a new line of genetic diversity to the captive population.

Kidogo—Willie B.'s only son, born in 1998—has the official name Willie B. Jr. *Kidogo* means "junior" in Swahili, the language spoken in the part of Africa from which Willie B. came. The zoo anticipates that as Kidogo gets older, more people will call him his given name to honor his famous dad. Like all gorillas, Kidogo is a vegetarian. He eats a variety of fruits and vegetables, branches, and leaves and gets extra vitamins and nutrients from specially formulated primate nuggets.

In the wild gorillas may live thirty to forty years, but in captivity they can live more than fifty years. Right now, though, Willie B. Jr. is just busy being a kid who enjoys wrestling with one of his sisters.

➤Bear right and pass the Muntijac otters' pond on the left.

➤Turn left at the dead end, which takes you to the Ketambe area, home of the orangutan. The orangutan feeding takes place at 2:30 and 2:45 P.M. daily.

➤Bear right and come to the World of Reptiles at the dead end to view one of the largest reptile exhibits in the Southeast.

➤Retrace your steps and turn left to go down the steps to the panda exhibit.

Of Interest

Lun Lun and Yang Yang

Pandas are among the rarest and most popular mammals in the world, with fewer than 1,000 in the wild and 200 in captivity. Lun Lun, a female, and Yang Yang, a male, came here from China in the fall of 1999. They had traveled 7,526 miles from Beijing, ending a fifteen-year quest to bring giant pandas here. President Jimmy Carter, a native Georgian, used his influence to help achieve this goal.

People call pandas bears, but scientists believe they are more closely related to raccoons. Chinese and American scientists have been working together for years, and they will trade information, hoping to save giant pandas from extinction. The animals will actually be on loan from China for ten years. About 120 giant pandas now live in captivity, but visitors may see only three others at U.S. zoos: two in San Diego and one in Washington.

The pandas weigh about 100 pounds each and will weigh about 165 to 350 pounds when adults. They measure 4 to 5 feet from nose to rump. They eat primarily bamboo and must eat about sixteen hours a day, eating twenty to forty pounds of food. That's a lot of bamboo! They are finicky eaters, often changing which type of bamboo they will eat. Zoo employees and volunteers scour the Atlanta area looking for bamboo—from the wild and from private gardens.

Architects who designed the $7-million indoor and outdoor panda habitat chose primarily conifers and bamboo, the flora one would find in the pandas' native environment. The plantings give the impression of visiting a Chinese forest. Large trees give the pandas shade. The habitat has many unique features to keep Lun Lun and Yang Yang active and content.

A Chinese-style shop—Pandamonium—near the panda habitat has all kinds of "panda" gifts.

You may watch the pandas eat, sleep, and play by logging onto www.accessatlanta.com/pandas.

➤Retrace your steps downhill and continue straight to see the tigers on the right. Loop back uphill to the left and bear right around the curve.

➤Turn right to enter the petting zoo. Continue past the wetlands and you will see exotic birds and lemurs as you continue downhill.

➤Children may take a ride on the carousel.

➤To ride the train walk behind the carousel to the train station.

➤Continue past the playground to the entrance and to the end of the walk.

The Atlanta Cyclorama

In Grant Park you will stroll along gentle walking paths and carriage roads through wooded land. Colonel Lemuel P. Grant, an engineer from New Hampshire who planned Atlanta's Civil War fortifications in 1863, donated eighty-five acres for the park. An additional forty-four acres increased its total size to 129 acres.

The Cyclorama stands at the center of the park in a 1921 neoclassical structure covered in terra-cotta. It contains the world's largest painting, the *Battle of Atlanta*.

This canvas, depicted in a round, measures 42 feet in height and 400 feet in circumference and revolves around a seated audience. The figures in the foreground, called a diorama, were added by WPA workers in 1936. The diorama blends perfectly with the painting to create a three-dimensional effect with terrain features like hills, ravine, shell-blasted stumps, wagons, and fighting men. It also includes a figure with the face of Clark Gable, who actually viewed the painting. Visitors cannot tell where the painting ends and the diorama begins. Through narration, music, and sound effects, history comes alive and takes visitors back to a hot day, July 22, 1864, to become part of the battle.

The battle was actually one of a series of Civil War engagements—known as the Atlanta Campaign—fought from May to September 1864. On the morning of July 22, Major General William T. Sherman and his Union troops encircled Atlanta. Confederate troops, under the command of General John B. Hood, attacked the Union armies in a desperate attempt to save Atlanta. The union troops defeated the Confederates. The painting depicts the beginning of this successful Union attack. Nightfall found more than 12,000 Americans dead, wounded, or missing.

A cyclorama is a large cylindrical painting that gained in popularity following the Civil War. Eleven meticulous German and Polish artists came to Atlanta in 1884 and researched the Battle of Atlanta to execute this painting. The completed work toured the country until an Atlantan bought it in 1892. It has been in its present location since 1921.

The *Texas,* one of the steam locomotives used in the Great Locomotive Chase in April 1862, dominates the main floor. A nearby display describes the chase—also known as Andrews' Raid—which began at Kennesaw, Georgia, when Union soldiers seized a locomotive called the *General.* Confederates on the *Texas* pursued the *General* north until they abandoned it near Ringgold, Georgia. The *Texas* has been a popular attraction in the Cyclorama since 1927. You can see the stolen train at the Kennesaw Historical Museum in Walk 16. You can also visit the historic hotel in Marietta where Andrews' Raiders spent the night before hijacking the *General* on the same walk.

The bookstore offers a wide range of Civil War replicas, memorabilia, and books on topics from military strategies to recipes from the 1800s.

The two-story building also contains a museum with a fascinating collection of Civil War artifacts, weapons, displays, maps, and photographs. Foreign visitors may secure audio multilingual translations of the Battle of Atlanta narrative.

Walk 6

Piedmont Park and the Atlanta Botanical Garden

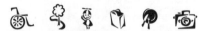

General location: These walks begin 2 miles northeast of downtown Atlanta.

Special attractions: Atlanta's second-largest and best-known public park and an outstanding botanical garden.

Difficulty rating: Mostly flat; all paved route.

Distance: 1.4 miles through Piedmont Park, 0.8 mile through the Botanical Garden.

Estimated time: 45 minutes through the park, 20 minutes through the garden.

Walk 6

Piedmont Park

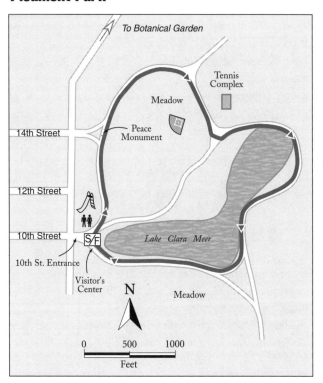

To Botanical Garden

Tennis Complex

Meadow

Peace Monument

14th Street

12th Street

10th Street

10th St. Entrance

Visitor's Center

S/F

Lake Clara Meer

N

Meadow

0   500   1000
Feet

Services: Rest rooms, restaurant, gift shop, water fountain, and soft-drink machine are available in the Botanical Garden. All areas of the garden are handicapped accessible, and you may request a wheelchair. Visitors may request an audiotape tour of the Conservatory in English, French, German, Spanish, and Japanese at the admissions booth.

Restrictions: Dogs must be on leashes no longer than 6 feet, and their droppings must be picked up in the park. Walk on designated pathways in the park. At the Botanical Garden visitors may take strollers in the outdoor gardens but must leave them outside when they enter the Conservatory. The garden bans smoking.

For more information: Call Piedmont Park and the Atlanta Botanical Garden.

Getting started: To reach this area from I–75 South, take exit 250, cross Tenth Street, and turn right onto Fourteenth Street. Cross Spring, West Peachtree, and Peachtree Streets. Fourteenth Street dead-ends at Piedmont Park on Piedmont Avenue; turn right to find the entrance for the park at Twelfth Street. You may park at the Colony Square complex after you cross Peachtree Street or in the lot past Colony Square. To find parking along side streets, turn left onto Piedmont; then turn left onto North Prado. To reach the Atlanta Botanical Garden, turn left at the dead end at Fourteenth and Piedmont, and then turn right at the first light on Prado. The garden has its own free parking with purchase of a ticket.

Public transportation: Regular MARTA buses run along Piedmont Avenue. The number 36 North Decatur bus runs from the Arts Center station. On Sunday take the number 31 Lindbergh bus from MARTA's Five Points or Lindbergh stations. The Arts Center station on Fifteenth Street behind the Woodruff Arts Center is within walking distance of the park. As you exit the station, turn left and walk uphill, cross Lombardy Way, and then cross Peachtree Street. Cross the street and follow that sidewalk on the right until it dead-ends into Piedmont Avenue. Turn right until you come to the park entrance on the left at Fourteenth Street. Call MARTA for current schedules, and confirm the bus's destination when you buy the ticket.

Walk 6

Overview: This walk begins at the 185-acre Piedmont Park, one of Atlanta's oldest. For more than one hundred years, Atlantans have gathered in the heart of the city for recreation, as well as for cultural and sports events. The park has served as a showplace for art, music, and politics, and as an anchor to surrounding neighborhoods. It is presently undergoing a $21.6-million face-lift.

Piedmont Park is one of the most heavily visited parks in the southeast United States. Approximately two million people visit it annually. There are paved trails for walking, bicycling, roller skating, and in-line skating. A 3-mile jogging trail, a lake, picnic sites, sports fields, and thirteen tennis courts round out the recreational opportunities. Children will enjoy the unusual playground, Playscapes.

Atlantans were not the first visitors to come to this plot of land. Muscogee Indians lived on this land originally, and white Georgia residents secured the land by drawing lots in the 1830s. The man who drew the winning ticket for this property sold it—along with a mill on Clear Creek—for $450 to Benjamin Walker. Walker and his wife built a log cabin, cleared the land, and farmed the 189 acres. Their son was born in the cabin. During the Civil War, Benjamin Walker enlisted in the Confederate army, and his family evacuated the property. After the war the Walkers found a devastated farm, but they rebuilt it even better than before.

By 1887 the city had started to spread out. A group of powerful, wealthy city leaders bought the Walker farm to start an exclusive club and park for horse enthusiasts. They called it the Gentlemen's Driving Club and built a racetrack for horse-and-buggy races. Seeing the money-making potential of this space, they organized the Piedmont Exposition Company.

The development of the park served as a magnet for streetcar lines, new streets, and residential growth. One thousand men built a main building, a new clubhouse, a grandstand for the racetrack, etc.

The first fair—the 1895 Piedmont Exposition—attracted 50,000 people and promoted the city's post–Civil War growth. In 1894 the city bought the park, but the Gentlemen's Driving Club remained under private ownership.

Piedmont Park and the Botanical Garden, adjacent to the park, are on the national Register of Historic Places.

Now start walking. The natural beauty of trails, trees, open space, and water await you.

The Walk

➤Your walk starts at the Piedmont Park Visitor's Center, which originally served as a women's comfort station in 1911.

➤Take the street to the left, past the playground. The stone urn and banisters outside the present banister on the steps on the left—built to last three months for the 1895 Exposition—still stand firm. The steps lead to the playground, one of only two such playscapes in the world. The other is in Kyoto, Japan. Isamu Noguchi, a Japanese-American sculptor, conceived and designed playgrounds so that children could learn abstract art by touching and climbing on everything.

➤As you continue walking, look up to the left and see the Peace Monument.

➤You will pass the meadow on the right. On the left you will see the Piedmont Driving Club, built around the

Walk 6

The Peace Monument

The figures in the sculpture symbolize the coming together of the North and South after the Civil War.

By the late 1870s Atlantans had endured nearly twenty years of hard times. They had to rebuild their city after The War between the States; then they underwent years of military occupation, called Reconstruction. Passions slowly cooled, however, and in 1877 President Rutherford B. Hayes withdrew the last federal troops from the South.

The Gate City Guard had been the first military company in Atlanta to volunteer for the war. Reactivated afterward, they decided to be the first to hold the peace. The guard proposed a "Peace Mission" to the northern states in 1879. They said, "The war is over; now it is time for peace."

During the next decades, other visits took place between Northerners and Southerners. In 1910 private subscriptions raised money to erect a monument to that first Northern Mission.

original farmhouse on the property. Margaret Mitchell, author of *Gone With the Wind*, used to drink martinis there out of a quart Mason canning jar that she brought from home.

➤Steps on the left, built for the 1895 Expo, lead to the Atlanta Botanical Garden. The garden leases its land from the park. Developers of the Expo cut 20 feet off the top of the hill to make space for the garden.

➤At the fork in the road, walk downhill to the right. At the bottom of the hill, walk straight to the sidewalk; turn left and start walking around Lake Clara Meer. The name means "Clear Lake" in Dutch.

➤When you reach the bridge to the left, you might want to walk there and look to the right to view the new areas of the park. Clear Creek originally ran under the bridge; by the 1970s, however, the creek had turned into a swamp. The new walkways that you see follow the design of Frederick Law Olmsted, the father of American landscape architecture.

Notice the plaque commemorating hoo-hoo trees planted by the Hoo-Hoo Club, a lumbermen's fraternal order. No one knows what a hoo-hoo tree is.

➤Continue walking beside the meadow on the left. Look for the painted orange line on the pavement, which marks the finish line for runners in the annual July Fourth Peachtree Race. On the left you will then walk past a hill where children go sledding when Atlanta has one of its infrequent snows.

Continue until you reach the Visitor's Center and the end of the walk.

The Atlanta Botanical Garden

Overview: The Atlanta Botanical Garden, founded in 1976, nestles among the towering office buildings and historic neighbors of midtown Atlanta. Flowers and wildlife create an oasis of fragrance and color in the smallest and youngest botanical gardens in the nation.

The thirty-three-acre sanctuary includes rose, fragrance, and herb gardens; fountains; a wooded overlook;

The Atlanta Botanical Garden

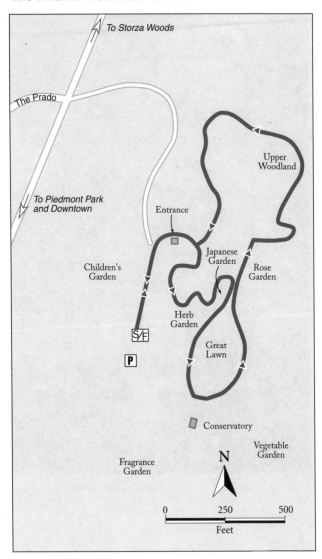

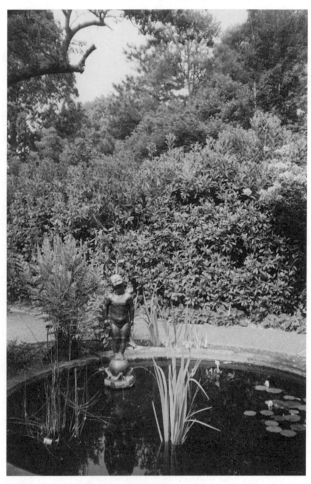

The Atlanta Botanical Garden features a number of statues and ponds.

and fifteen acres of outdoor displays. The garden has two wooded areas. The Upper Woodland has five lush, shady acres filled with wildflowers, ferns, and plants native to Georgia. Storza Woods, a fifteen-acre hardwood forest—one of the few remaining in Atlanta—has walking trails. The $5.5-million, glass-enclosed Dorothy Chapman Fuque Conservatory has an outstanding collection of more than 7,000 rare and endangered orchids, as well as tropical, desert, and Old World plants.

The garden leads the world in the study of carnivorous plants, spearheading efforts to preserve endangered species. Highly trained staff members use a tissue-culture laboratory to propagate plants as well as new cultivars for the trade. They accept and care for illegally imported plants confiscated by the government, and they identify and maintain plant populations in the world. They rate new plant selections for hardiness, disease resistance, and length of bloom period in the outdoor gardens. The best performers appear in the spring and fall members-only plant sale catalogs.

The garden's outstanding Conservation Program focuses on regionally and internationally endangered plant species.

In the fall of 1999, the garden, in conjunction with the Scottish Rite Children's Hospital, opened Atlanta's first garden designed just for children. Children enter this imaginative garden by way of a unique flower bridge. Water features, a child-sized maze, an outdoor amphitheater, a dinosaur garden where they can dig for "fossils," a tree house, and much more thrill them.

The Museum Shop offers gifts with a botanical flair.

The Walk

➤Start the walk at the parking lot. You may enter the Children's Garden on the left across from the entrance. As you walk toward the admissions booth, look on the right for the Glory Border, which features perennials and new introductions to the trade. Pick up a map when you buy your ticket. Enter the courtyard; then bear right. The hanging greenery that disguises the building creates a natural setting.

➤Take a right exit and walk to the right, where you'll see a tall Chinese chestnut tree. Chinese chestnuts remained immune to the blight that killed American chestnut trees during the 1930s.

Look to the left to see the Lotus Fountain. Notice the figures under the waterfall and the lotus flowers and leaves around the sides. The artist makes tiles in her home and then constructs the fountains at different locations.

➤As you walk to the right, you will see the back side of the Glory Border and, on the left, an area of mixed shrubs. Notice the *Frog Baby* statue in the pond. The High Museum has placed some sculptures on permanent loan to the garden. Look for two statues—one of St. Francis of Assisi and one of a piper—as you walk.

➤Bear left, past the Iris Garden, which blooms in spring.

➤Turn right to enter the Herb Garden through the wrought-iron gate that has garden tools built into its design. This garden serves a teaching purpose as well as for pleasure. The herbs on the right offer fragrance and use as beverages. Culinary herbs line the area on the right wall. Medicinal herbs that Indians used line the area along the far wall. Boxwoods divide the sections. Visitors are encouraged to pick and smell the leaves.

The Princess Tree

The tallest tree behind the *Frog Baby* statue is the paulownia (pronounced paw-low-nee-uh), nicknamed the Princess tree, a China native used to make furniture. According to Chinese legend, a father planted a paulownia tree at a baby girl's birth. When the daughter married, her father chopped down the tree and made her a hope chest in which to store her best clothing. The highly fire-resistant wood protected the clothing even when straw houses burned.

The tree was used in folk medicine in rural China to remedy graying hair, fever, and liver ailments. By the eleventh century monks in Buddhist monasteries used the wood for dishes and coffins.

The pale-colored wood was first imported into Europe in the 1830s. It got its nickname from Princess Anna Pavlovna, wife of Prince Wilhelm of the Netherlands and granddaughter of Catherine the Great of Russia.

The trees, the world's fastest-growing, were introduced in the United States in about 1850, possibly from seeds mixed in with packing material from Asia. Now there are approximately 10,000 acres grown commercially. The wood is used to make furniture and musical instruments such as violins and dulcimers, as well as plywood and molding. Paulownia wood is second only to black cherry in price.

The American Paulownia Association tries to spread the popularity of the tree. The wood doesn't shrink, you can drive nails into it and it doesn't split, and it's very light but relatively strong. At this time, there is not enough public demand for a lumber company to stock it.

People usually look on this tree as a "trash" tree because birds scatter the seeds widely, and they often wind up having an unwanted tree.

➤Leave the Herb Garden and bear right to reach the Shade Garden, which consists mostly of hydrangeas.

➤Walk across the pathway to enter the Japanese Garden.

➤Exit the Japanese garden and turn right on the allée, arched by white Natchez crape myrtles.

➤Bear right at the water fountain. You will pass a semi-circular stone bench monument on the right that the family of Ann Lyon Crammond, the Atlanta Botanical Garden's first director, donated. All those presently connected with the garden say that every flower that comes up is a monument to her.

➤Walk under the vine arbor beside the Nursery and Greenhouses—closed to the public—and the $1.5 million state-of-the-art support greenhouse.

Of Interest

Safe from Evil Spirits

A hurricane destroyed much of the original Japanese Garden, and a local Japanese carpenter re-created it authentically. The Bank of Kygoshima—located in Atlanta's sister city—donated the 300-year-old lantern on the left.

Greenery predominates: different shades and shapes of leaves, pruned pine trees, and only a few long-limbed plants. Japanese gardens have few flowers because the Japanese feel that dying flowers cause sadness. Other elements include running water, goldfish, pebbles, large stones that represent the continents, a bridge, and a lamp.

The round moon-gate on the left is of Chinese origin. Walkways in Japanese gardens curve, to keep out evil spirits, who can only move in straight lines.

As you near the Conservatory, you will see on the right the Hearty Palm section with Burmese palms and Chinese fan fronds. The Lily Pond is directly in front of the building.

➤If you want to visit the vegetable gardens and the Fragrance Garden for the Visually Impaired, you will find them behind the Conservatory. An iron rail leads visually handicapped people around the circle, past an area dedicated to perennials. This special garden enables people to touch, taste, and smell the herbs even if they cannot see them.

➤Bear left around the green space. You will go by an area dedicated to perennials.

Of Interest

Dorothy Chapman Fuque Conservatory

Orchids bloom here year-round. The Conservatory has the largest orchid collection in the Southeast outside of Florida, as well as many rare species not seen elsewhere. A Tropical Forest has plants of every description, exotic birds, and gecko lizards.

The sequence of the displays follows the plants' order of appearance on the planet. First come the ferns, the cycads section that contain cone-bearing plants, the first seed-bearing plants section, and begonias. The Conservatory also has one of the top collections of Old World palms in the United States.

The Desert House features plants that come from Europe, Asia, and Africa.

The Conservatory is wheelchair accessible.

➤Retrace your steps through the allée, pass the Lanier Terrace, and walk up the steps at the end. Bear right and pass the Wildflower Garden. You will enjoy *Isobel,* a statue of a child crossing a stream.

➤The ceiling of the Alston Lookout shows the four seasons Atlanta enjoys.

➤Walk downhill to the right through the Woodland Rockery and pass the Hosta Gardens on the hill behind the rockery.

➤Walk uphill and go down the steps. Enter the building to return to the entrance and the end of the walk.

Walk 7
Freedom Path

    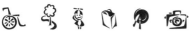

General location: 5 minutes from downtown.

Special attractions: Hiking trail, Carter Presidential Center with beautiful gardens.

Difficulty rating: Moderate; hilly; all on sidewalks.

Distance: 2.4 miles.

Estimated time: 1 hour, 10 minutes.

Services: Cafe open for lunch; rest rooms available in Carter Center; a museum store; wheelchairs available at the library; free parking.

Restrictions: Dogs must be on leashes no longer than 6 feet, and their droppings must be picked up. The museum charges admission.

For more information: Call the Atlanta Convention and Visitors Bureau and the Carter Presidential Center.

Freedom Path

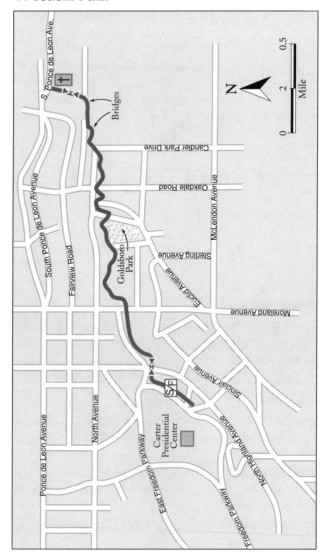

Walk 7

Getting started: From the north or south, take I–75/85 to Freedom Parkway. Take exit 248C and follow signs to the Carter Center for 1.8 miles. From downtown go east on North Avenue for approximately 1.5 miles to Freedom Parkway. Turn right onto Highway E42. The Carter Center, with free parking, is on the left.

Public transportation: Take MARTA bus route 16 Noble. Call MARTA for current schedules, and confirm the bus's destination when you buy the ticket.

Overview: Freedom Path came about when the persistent opposition of Atlanta home owners killed plans for three multilane roads. As a result in-town neighborhoods were preserved and space was opened for the city's largest park. The Freedom Park Conservancy has raised millions of dollars to transform 207 acres cleared of 500 homes into a park. It took two separate, bitter road wars to achieve this.

In the mid-1960s, the Department of Transportation (DOT) began condemning land for two highways that would have sliced through some of east Atlanta's most historic neighborhoods. Years of aggressive neighborhood opposition persuaded then-Gov. Jimmy Carter to kill the plan in 1972. But acres of land—cleared and still owned by the DOT—remained, and the respite for these neighborhoods from fighting roads would be short-lived. In the early 1980s one of the proposed highways was revived in the form of the Presidential Parkway, intending to connect downtown with Carter's presidential library. A new corps of opponents formed, reinforced by many veterans of the earlier fight. They held countless rallies and protests; some were arrested trying to block bulldozers and chainsaws from pushing over trees. They also took their fight to court, and the project was delayed. After almost a decade,

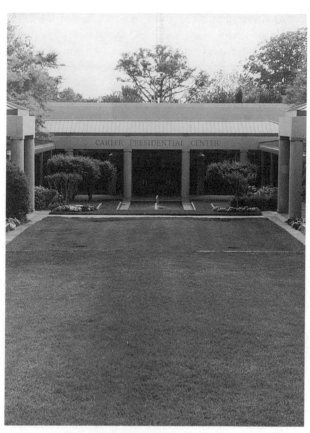

The Carter Presidential Center includes gardens, a wildflower meadow, a cherry orchard, waterfalls, and two small lakes in a thirty-five-acre park. (Courtesy Jimmy Carter Library; David Stanhope, photographer)

the groups compromised, producing the present-day Freedom Parkway, a shortened, landscaped boulevard lined with jogging trails.

The Carter Presidential Center lies at the heart of the four legs of Freedom Path in a thirty-five-acre park. The grounds include formal gardens, a wildflower meadow, a cherry orchard, and waterfalls tucked between two small lakes. The Rose Garden has 400 plants and eighty varieties, including the coral Rosalynn Carter rose. The serene Japanese garden—designed by Master Gardener Kinsaku Nakane—includes river birch, golden raintree, Japanese maples, camellias, azaleas, and rhododendrons.

Jimmy and Rosalynn Carter established the nonprofit Carter Center, a unique blend of history and history in the making. In partnership with Emory University, the center seeks to prevent and resolve conflicts, enhance freedom and democracy, and improve health worldwide. "We work alongside the world's forgotten people—those who are the most in need and underserved," says former President Jimmy Carter.

Next door the Jimmy Carter Museum offers visitors an intimate look at the American presidency, important events of the twentieth century, and the Carter administration.

Highlights include a film on the evolution of the office of president, reproductions of the inaugural gowns worn by previous first ladies, and a replica of the Oval Office. Visitors will also see a formal dinner setting from the White House and memorabilia from President Carter's 1976 campaign. In an interactive video of a Jimmy Carter "Town Hall" meeting, visitors can ask questions of the former president.

The Jimmy Carter Library—the only presidential library in the Southeast—located beside the museum, provides a rich resource for students and scholars of American history. Open by appointment, the archives cover the Carter administration from foreign and domestic policy to daily life in the White House.

The Walk

You will walk the east-west leg of Freedom Path within the park. The westernmost end of the park touches the Martin Luther King Jr. Historic District. You can read about that district in Walk 3.

►Start at the upper (south) side of the museum across Highway E42, which becomes East Freedom Parkway, and turn left. The park's trails wind through some of Atlanta's oldest neighborhoods including Inman Park, the city's first suburb, on the right. You can read about that neighborhood in Walk 9.

►Cross North Highland Avenue. You are walking through an area where Union troops camped—overlooking what is now downtown—during the Battle of Atlanta in 1864 during the Civil War.

►Cross Moreland Avenue. At this point you might want to walk 1 block to the right to Little Five Points, a diverse artistic center with theaters, restaurants, and shops.

As you continue, you will first pass the Candler Park neighborhood on the left and then the Druid Hills neighborhood. You may read about that neighborhood in Walk 10.

As you reach the highest point on the trail, you are standing on Goldsboro Hill. Notice the trees—white oak, water oak, pecan, and tulip poplar—some 150 years old. Goldsboro Park has tennis and basketball courts.

➤Cross Euclid Avenue. You will see people rollerblade, jog, bike, and walk here. Freedom Park is unique because of its skinny X-shape, which attracts more in-line skaters than picnicking families.

➤Cross Oakdale Road.

➤When you reach the point where North Avenue and Candler Park Drive join, walk across the street and continue downhill.

➤Cross the bridge over the west tributary of Lullwater Creek.

➤Cross the second bridge over the creek.

➤Turn left when you reach the church and walk to South Ponce de Leon Avenue. The people who opposed the Presidential Parkway climbed the 150-year-old trees on the church's front lawn and in Shadyside Park across the street during the protests to prevent their being cut.

Look to the left across the bridge on Ponce de Leon to see the beginning of the Druid Hills neighborhood. If you walk 1/4 mile to the right, you would reach Clifton Avenue. The Fernbank Museum—mentioned in Walk 14—is downhill on the left on Clifton.

➤Retrace your steps and return to the starting point.

Walk 8
Ansley Park

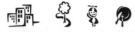

General location: This area lies 15 blocks north of the downtown Atlanta area.

Special attractions: Winding streets, picturesque parks, outstanding architecture, historic churches, and the Robert W. Woodruff Arts Center, which includes the High Museum of Art.

Difficulty rating: Easy; mostly flat; and entirely on sidewalks. Some of the sidewalks are set with hexagonal stones, an Atlanta tradition. Exercise some caution if walking in narrow heels and keep an eye out for tree roots.

Distance: 1 mile.

Estimated time: 30 minutes.

Services: Restaurants and rest rooms are available in Colony Square; rest rooms are available in the Arts Center.

Ansley Park

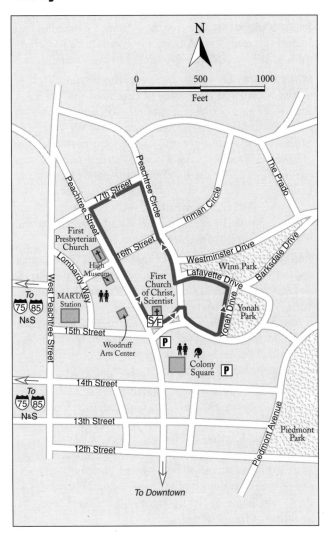

Restrictions: Dogs must be on leashes no longer than 6 feet, and their droppings must be picked up.

For more information: Contact the Atlanta Convention and Visitors Bureau. The Atlanta Preservation Center offers tours of this area March–November.

Getting started: This walk begins at the First Church of Christ Scientist at the corner of Peachtree and Fifteenth Streets. From I–75 North, take exit 250 and turn left at Fourteenth. Go 3 blocks and turn left onto Peachtree Street. To park turn right into Colony Square's Garage, or go straight through the light on Peachtree Street and turn left into lots under the hotel or to the public lot past the hotel.

From I–75 South, take exit 249—the Fourteenth–Tenth Streets exit—and turn right onto Fourteenth. Follow the directions above to Peachtree Street.

Public transportation: MARTA buses number 10 Peachtree and number 23 Lenox/Arts run along Peachtree Street, and the number 35 Ansley Park circles through the neighborhood from the Arts Center station, which is adjacent to the Woodruff Arts Center on Fifteenth Street. Call MARTA for current schedules and confirm the bus's destination when you buy the ticket.

Overview: You will meander through an area filled with aesthetic delights. Many parks, placed along streams and in dales, give the neighborhood a pastoral flavor. The entire development, which is filled with elegant, old homes, is on the National Register of Historic Places.

Ansley Park became Atlanta's first automobile suburb, so-called because automobile owners, no longer dependent on public transportation, lived there. This suburb is the first example of "white flight" from a downtown the wealthy had found undesirable.

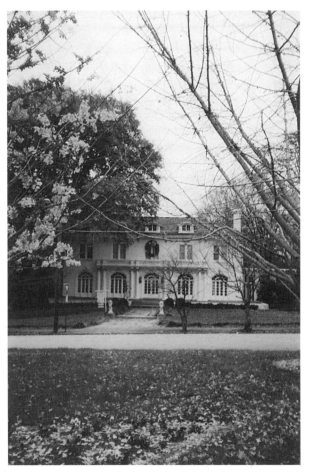

*Ansley Park contains some of Atlanta's most elegant, old homes. The
entire development is on the National Register of Historic Places.*

Atlanta first developed around the Five Points area—where Peachtree, Marietta, Decatur, and Edgewood Streets converge—and wealthy people built big homes there. As Five Points began to turn commercial, the home owners wanted to move out of that area. In 1904 developer Edwin P. Ansley responded to their need and promised a "white suburb." Three *A*s enabled Ansley Park to develop: affluence, attitude, and, later, automobiles. Ansley bought a 350-acre family estate. Solon Z. Ruff, a civil engineer who had worked on the first plans for Druid Hills with Frederick Law Olmsted, developed the neighborhood. Ansley built broad streets he called "driving boulevards." Ruff razed the original trees; the present trees, which add much to the neighborhood's beauty, grew later.

The Model-T Ford came out in 1910, and in five years Ansley Park residents owned half of all the cars in Atlanta. In 1909 only 16 percent of Atlanta's social register lived in Ansley Park; by 1926, 74 percent lived there.

Atlantans consider Ansley Park the worst place to get lost in the entire city, as the area has no evident pattern to the winding streets, no straight avenues, and no square blocks. Since Ansley built this development for car drivers, he did not need straight streets suitable for streetcars. The story goes that in the park's early days a man took a cat far from home, hoping to lose it. In the end the man got lost and had to follow his cat back home!

Now start walking on a trek that will delight you every step of the way.

The Walk

➤Start at the First Church of Christ Scientist at the corner of Peachtree Street and Fifteenth Street. This 1913 building is one of the few neoclassical buildings in Atlanta, and its copper dome has long been an Atlanta landmark.

Look across Fifteenth Street to see Colony Square, the Southeast's first multiuse high rise. The complex contains town houses, offices, boutiques, a food court and restaurants, rest rooms, and the 500-room Colony Square Hotel.

►Walk downhill on Fifteenth Street. On the right you will see tiny Ansley Park, which Hattie High donated in honor of the Daughters of the American Revolution. (The High Museum, a site on this walk, bears her husband's name.)

►Cross Peachtree Circle at the crosswalk. Look downhill to the house at number 24 on the left, one of Ansley Park's earliest houses, a renovated 1905 Queen Anne style.

►Turn right and walk uphill. At One Peachtree Circle, on your left, you will pass an Italianate villa designed by popular architect Walter Thomas Downing. Notice the five large French doors across the front and the two sculptured lions at the entrance. A previous owner once had difficulty trying to describe to a painter that she wanted the exterior painted its present color, sunset rose. The painter replied dryly, "Oh, you mean pink."

At 178 Fifteenth you will find the oldest house in Ansley Park. Architect Alexander C. Bryant designed the Romanesque house that imitates the Victorian style.

The noted Atlanta architect Neel Reid designed the Georgian house at 186 Fifteenth Street. He supposedly designed houses while thinking of an Italian villa. He built garages with upstairs apartments behind the homes because one family in six had servants.

►Turn left onto Yonah Drive at the corner. You will see Yonah Park on the right, one of Ansley Park's many green spaces.

➤At the bottom of the hill, turn left onto LaFayette Drive. You will be walking beside Winn Park on the right.

At 31 LaFayette Drive you will see the home of P. Thornton Marye, the architect who designed the Fox Theater, which you will see on Walk 11. Marye imported all the materials for this Italian-style villa from Italy. The villa—with its many tall doors and windows that allowed for good air circulation—suited the Atlanta climate beautifully since homes did not have air conditioning.

As you dead-end at Peachtree Circle, you may want to spend some time in Winn Park. The greenery, a stream, and benches make it a pleasant spot.

➤Cross Peachtree Circle and turn right.

The 1920 house at 68 Peachtree Circle reflects the Frank Lloyd Wright Prairie-style architecture. The 1948 one-story neoclassical-style house at number 72 is rare because that style usually had two stories. The 1917 Neel Reid neocolonial house at number 107 shows how Reid made a small house look impressive.

The California-style bungalow at 126 Peachtree Circle gives an example of a house that became popular in Ansley Park in the 1920s. This style was built to look older on the outside, and the insides have beautiful woodwork and built-in cabinets. The Neel Reid house at number 132 sold for nearly $1 million in 1998.

At the corner of Seventeenth Street, look on the hill on the right to the site of an old girls' school, Woodberry Hall. The first woman who entered the University of Georgia built this school, and Margaret Mitchell attended there. The 1858 Ionic columns came from a downtown residence.

➤Turn left onto Seventeenth Street. The large apartment at the corner exemplifies a trend in the 1920s, when builders designed apartment buildings to look like single-family dwellings from the front.

►When you reach Peachtree Street, look to the right at the second building from the corner, number 1401. It rests on the site of the house where Margaret Mitchell lived during her adolescence. Mitchell's mother achieved her dream that the family have a home on Peachtree Street. Mitchell did not like the house, however, and in her will, she stipulated that her brother, Stephens, destroy that house.

Look straight downhill on Seventeenth. Margaret Mitchell and her husband, John Marsh, lived on the first floor of the Russell Apartments on this site from 1932 to 1939. She finished writing *Gone With the Wind* there. The apartments have since been torn down.

►Turn left onto Peachtree Street. Across the street at number 1382, you will face one of the four original homes built in Atlanta. This sandstone brick house has features reminiscent of the Tudor Revival style. An architectural firm now occupies the building.

►You will pass Reid House, the Georgian-Eclectic–style apartment building designed by Philip Shutze and Hal Hertz, members of noted Atlanta architect Neel Reid's firm. The building started out as a luxury apartment house, only the third such in the city.

Across the street you will see the First Presbyterian Church, a neo-Gothic sandstone structure noted Atlantan Walter Thomas Downing designed in 1919. The stained-glass windows were made by the Tiffany Studio of New York and the D'Ascenzo Studios of Philadelphia. This church broadcast the first religious services in the South in 1922.

►Cross Sixteenth. The High Museum across the street is part of the Robert W. Woodruff Arts Center and is the centerpiece of Atlanta's Midtown Arts District. The museum, which opened in 1984, bears the name of Joseph M. High. His widow, wealthy Harriett (Hattie) High, donated the property for the original museum. Architect Richard Meier designed the building, which has received numerous architectural awards.

The museum displays European and American paintings and sculptures. It also has outstanding collections of African, decorative, and twentieth-century art as well as photographs and graphics. The gallery About Masks provides fun for kids of all ages.

On the lawn you will see a bronze casting of Auguste Rodin's *L'Ombre*, "The Shade." The French government

Of Interest

Controversy at the High

In 1969 the High Museum hosted its annual Southeastern Annual Exhibition. The exhibition included a nude called *Go-Go-Girl* by Frank Rampolla. Nudes had hung in the museum before, but some board members objected to one hanging in the main lobby, a space children visited.

The director removed the nude, and some people protested. *Atlanta Constitution* columnist Harold Martin jokingly said that the main problem came not from the painting's eroticism, but rather, from the subject's being just plain ugly. She was "a sclerotic-looking old bag of bones of some 40 summers, who obviously has eaten too many starchy foods and avoided all forms of exercise," he wrote. "It couldn't be obscene because this picture wouldn't arouse a prurient interest in the bosom of a sailor just back from a three-year whaling voyage."

The director of the High hung the lady on his office walls and invited all lookers to see her there.

presented it to Atlanta in tribute to the victims of a plane crash at Orly Airport in Paris. In June 1962, 106 of Atlanta's most prominent patrons of the arts flew to visit European museums; tragically, the plane crashed, and all except the stewardesses died.

▶You next pass the main building of the Robert W. Woodruff Arts Center, home to the Alliance Theater, the Atlanta Symphony Orchestra, and the Atlanta College of Art. The Alliance Theater opened in 1969 and merged with the respected Atlanta Children's Theater in 1977. By the mid-1980s the Alliance ranked among the top ten resident theaters in America. The Atlanta Symphony Orchestra, begun in 1945, is among the country's most respected orchestras.

Of Interest

The Robert W. Woodruff Arts Center

In the 1950s and 1960s, Atlanta lacked first-class arts facilities. Robert W. Woodruff, head of Coca-Cola and the city's great philanthropist, gave $4 million to build an arts center.

Following the fatal plane crash at Orly Airport in 1962, the city's desire to establish a memorial to the dead merged with the plan to build an arts center. In 1968 the $13-million Atlanta Memorial Arts Center opened as the desired memorial. In 1979 Woodruff made the last large gift in his life, a $7.5-million grant for the new High Museum building. The Arts Alliance trustees named the complex after him.

For the first time in the United States, a large city fused visual arts, performing arts, and art education within a single institution.

➤At the corner of Peachtree Street and Fifteenth, look across the street to the right beside the AT&T building. A house people call The Castle represents the boyhood fantasies of eccentric owner Ferdinand McMillan, an agricultural machinery dealer. He built a medieval fortress of Stone Mountain granite, gray walls, and serrated top. He included narrow window slits to accommodate cannons and a turret, and called it Fort Peace. AT&T saved the house from the wrecking ball and renovated it, but it has sat idle for several years.

➤You have come to the end of the walk.

Walk 9

Inman Park

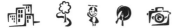

General location: About 2 miles east of downtown via Edgewood Avenue.

Special attractions: Large, ornate brightly painted Victorian homes on tree-lined avenues.

Difficulty rating: Easy; mostly flat, with one steep hill.

Distance: 1.6 miles.

Estimated time: 45 minutes.

Services: Restaurants with rest rooms for customers only. Free parking on streets.

Restrictions: Dogs must be on leashes no longer than 6 feet, and their droppings must be picked up.

For more information: Call the Atlanta Convention and Visitors Bureau.

Inman Park

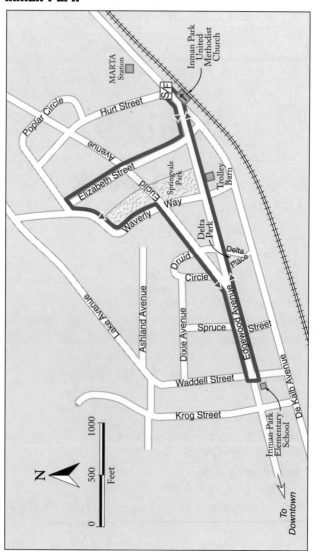

Walk 9

Getting started: When heading north or south on I–75/85, take exit 248C. Go 1.8 miles to the Carter Center. Continue and take a right on Highland Avenue, a left on Elizabeth Street, then a right on Edgewood. Drive to the MARTA station at the end of the street. You may park free on most side streets.

Public transportation: Inman Park–Reynoldstown MARTA is adjacent to DeKalb Avenue at Hurt Street. Regular bus service on route number 17 Decatur/Lakewood is available along Edgewood Avenue. Call MARTA for current schedules and confirm bus's destination when you buy the ticket.

Overview: As you walk the streets of Inman Park, you will step back in time to the late nineteenth century. Enough buildings of this romantic era remain together to give a distinct character to an entire residential area. You will see High Victorian, Queen Anne, late Victorian Colonial, and Classical Revival–style homes. The area is listed on the National Register of Historic Places.

During the Civil War, Union troops marched through this area. Some of the worst fighting took place on the eastern boundaries of the Inman Park area on July 22, 1864. You can see the painting of that battle in the Cyclorama painting in Grant Park in Walk 5.

After the war Atlanta moved toward building a diversified economy based not just on agriculture, but on manufacturing and industry. Joel Hurt, one of the city's leading developers, realized that Atlanta's lack of roads hampered its expansion to the east, so he planned a skyscraper at the downtown end of Edgewood Avenue and a trolley line connecting it to a garden suburb at the other end, 2 miles east. He started the city's first electric streetcar line, and the first in the country that ran on two rails. On August

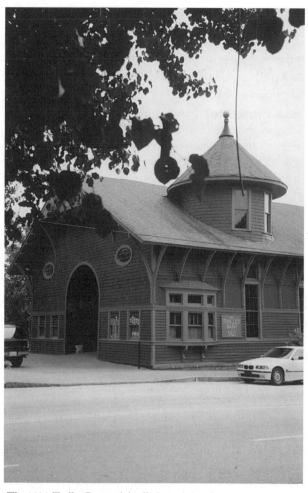

The 1890 Trolley Barn originally housed electric streetcars. Today it serves as a community center.

22, 1889, a yellow electric trolley with wooden benches made its first trip to the Trolley Barn at Inman Park. Even though the automobile later pushed the trolley into the shadows, the trolley greatly aided Atlanta's rapid expansion toward the suburbs.

Hurt created Inman Park, the first planned residential suburb. To do this he bought 189 acres of mostly farm land. The neighborhood would have a country feeling, yet provide all the conveniences of the city. He developed existing terrain, respecting native trees and plants, such as live oak trees. He named the neighborhood after his business associate and wealthy cotton merchant Samuel Inman. You can visit Inman's home, Swan House, on Walk 12.

Technological advances freed home builders from the square form, and rooms could have curves rather than corners, elements of Victorian architecture. Houses could have tall windows rather than the small panes of earlier years, as well as stained-glass windows. They had soaring brick chimneys and decorative porches. Families had hot and cold running water and electricity, among the first in Georgia to enjoy such amenities.

As you walk, look for homes built in the Queen Anne style. They usually have a wraparound porch and gingerbread and spindles around the porch; a tower; windows of different shapes and sizes; a decorative surface texture, such as fish-scale shingles; and an asymmetrical shape.

Hurt ran out of money before implementing all his ideas, so his dream did not come to full fruition. Cars enabled people to move farther out, and they no longer needed the streetcar. By 1920 people no longer found the out-of-date architecture fashionable.

The neighborhood went into a period of decline due to a housing shortage following World War I. The federal government paid home owners to subdivide their homes to provide housing for returning servicemen. The wealthier residents moved out, and blue-collar families moved in. The new families often lived in "shotgun" houses, so called because someone could stand at the front door and shoot straight through the house.

During the 1960s, absentee—and often negligent—landlords owned 70 percent of the homes, and renters did not modernize them. Some of the homes operated as 50-cents-a-night boardinghouses. In 1970 Robert Griggs and other concerned Inman Park residents formed Inman Park Restoration, Inc., sparking a restoration movement.

Now more than one hundred owners live in their own houses in the neighborhood. In 1973 the entire neighborhood received recognition as a historic district and was added to the National Register of Historic Places. At present a butterfly banner, symbol of the remarkable community efforts, hangs in windows of restored homes.

Now get walking to see the beauty from an earlier era. Mature trees give the area a pastoral charm.

The Walk

➤Begin at the corner of Edgewood Avenue and Hurt Street, heading away from MARTA. To the left, down Hurt, you will see three restaurants.

➤You will pass the Inman Park United Methodist Church, which Joel Hurt and his wife attended. The 1898 Stone Mountain granite building resembles an English parish church, with elements of the Romanesque Revival style.

➤Turn right on Elizabeth Street. At number 117 you will find the modest 1882 cottage where Hurt lived while developing the neighborhood. (The cottage was moved here from another location.) Hurt brought back plants from his travels and introduced the evergreen to Atlanta. The evergreen in the front yard is the only redwood of its kind documented east of the Mississippi River.

The Victorian–design house at number 127 has a true Victorian color scheme, showing the colors of nature.

At 132 Elizabeth you will see one of Leila Ross Wilburn's designs, a house built by and for a woman. This 1913 house has classical Ionic columns and a Craftsman overhanging roof with exposed rafters. The Craftsman style developed from 1910 through the 1930s as a reaction to the excessive ornamentation of the Victorian era. Craftsman bungalows typically have low, broad, gabled roofs that extend beyond the walls of the house.

Of Interest

Pioneering Southern Woman Architect

Leila Ross Wilburn became the South's second woman architect in 1909, when she opened her own business in downtown Atlanta at age 24.

It took Leila many difficult years to develop a clientele. But, she said, "This experience is compensated for today, however, by the pleasure which comes from building homes." She concluded, "There is nothing I like better, and I don't believe I'd be satisfied with any other job in the world."

Leila got her ideas by traveling from coast to coast, taking her sketchpad and camera with her. The time was ripe for her work. The South was recovering from the depressions of the late 1800s. Atlanta was experiencing a burst of growth with new buildings springing up everywhere. The banking and insurance industries required new buildings to house their growth. The people manning those fields needed homes, both within the city and in the suburbs.

Leila filled the needs more than adequately. Prior to this period, those with wealth built ostentatious Victorian homes. A growing middle-class responded positively to Leila's contrasting designs that offered functionality and efficient uses of every inch in the house. She described her designs as having "useful built-in furniture and artistic effects as bookcases, window seats, buffets, plate rails, concealed beds, ironing boards." She claimed that "being a woman, I feel I know the little things that should go into a house to make living in it a pleasure for the entire family." She advised builders to use plenty of windows, as "sunlight is cheaper than doctor bills."

Leila practiced architecture for 58 years until she died in 1967 at the age of 82. She achieved the distinction of being one of the pioneer women architects not only in Atlanta but in the entire South.

Bishop Warren Candler—brother of Asa Candler, the founder of Coca-Cola—lived in the simple 1910 Victorian house at number 144. Candler School of Theology at Emory University carries Bishop Candler's name.

At 145 Elizabeth you will pass Callan Castle, Asa Candler's home at that time. He named it after the family's ancestral home in Ireland. This 14,000-square-foot 1903 house, one of the largest in Inman Park, showed Candler's status. The white classical columns, typical of some pre–Civil War homes, had come back into style. The basement had a walk-in safe, where Candler kept the famous secret formula for Coca-Cola. Candler gave his Coca-Cola stock to his children and sold the company to Ernest

Walk 9

Woodruff. He and his wife later moved to Druid Hills. You can see that home on Walk 10.

➤Cross Euclid Avenue.

The 1904 Italianate house at 167 Elizabeth served as Joel Hurt's actual home, after he moved out of his cottage.

Number 177 is the first house built on the street.

Asa Candler had the house at number 182 specifically built to look like a hunting lodge in 1908.

The house at number 185 shows the best of Inman Park's Victorian architecture, an example of Steamboat Victorian. Notice the features not available before 1900, such as curving windows. The Civil War surgeon general had the house built in 1907.

Charles C. Candler, Asa's son, lived in the house at number 188. He served as president of Coca-Cola one year before Ernest Woodruff took over.

➤Turn left, cross Elizabeth, and walk downhill on Waverly Way.

The house at number 180 is one of two built for the manager of the Fulton Bag and Cotton Mill. You can read about the mill in Walk 4.

You will pass Springvale Park on the left. Euclid Avenue cut the park into half at the far end, and the park continues on the other side.

Neil Reed, famous Atlanta architect, built his only house in Inman Park at number 114. The Moorish-style house has shingle-style wood on the bottom, with shingles on top. During the Victorian period owners painted such houses two colors.

Howard Hirsch, an early Coca-Cola lawyer, lived at number 118. He got the company through some tough trade battles, and his actions kept the company in Atlanta.

At one time Asa Candler wanted to move the company to New York City, and the lawyer refused.

➤Turn right on Euclid Avenue.

Robert and Emily Woodruff spent their honeymoon in the house on the corner across the street at 100 Euclid. You will pass their first home at number 882. Woodruff bought the Coca-Cola Company from Asa Candler.

The bungalow at number 881 was built in the 1920s to 1940s.

Joel Hurt built the house at number 882 as a model house for his new community. A Swedish architect, Gottfried Norrman, designed the house. George Woodruff of

Of Interest

The House That Sparked Restoration Efforts

The house at 886 Euclid Avenue sparked the Inman Park restoration efforts in the 1960s. John M. Beath built this house, one of Inman Park's best, around 1890 for his Philadelphia bride. He promised his fiancée that if she came South, he would build her the finest home in Atlanta.

One day in the late 1950s, professional designer and architect Robert Griggs fell in love with the house—then in terrible shape. After fighting his way through the junk-strewn lawn, he found the woodwork and parquet floors in good shape in spite of years of neglect and overcrowding. Although everyone told him not to buy it, he paid $22,000 for it in 1969. He spent $50,000 to turn it from eight apartments back into a family dwelling.

This Queen Anne–style house features a rich display of materials: granite, brick, marble, slate, wood, wood shingles, terra-cotta, glass, and paint. It has no square rooms. Notice the pillars on the front porch and the pink marble.

Columbus, Georgia, bought it for his son Ernest and wife, Emily. Ernest Woodruff lived here for several years.

➤Cross both sides of Druid Circle.

➤Turn right on Edgewood Avenue where you'll find the Magnolia Bed & Breakfast at number 804. The Queen Anne–style house has a gazebo at the edge of the front porch.

➤Cross Spruce Street. Bishop Candler once lived in number 790 on the corner.

➤Cross Waddell Street.

➤Cross Edgewood. Look down the street to the right to see the 1892 Victorian red-brick Inman Park Elementary School, one of the earliest examples of Atlanta's school buildings, which also resembles college buildings of that period.

➤Retrace your steps on Edgewood and cross Waddell and Spruce.

➤Cross Delta Place. You will come to Delta Park, where you will see the Old Police Lock-up of 1880s vintage. Foot patrolmen locked one prisoner at a time in this "iron maiden" while waiting for the paddy wagon to pick him up to take him to jail.

➤Cross the other side of Delta Place.

The 1893 house at 814 Edgewood, a good example of the Eastlake–style house, still has its original stained-glass windows.

You will pass the King-Keith Bed & Breakfast at 889 Edgewood, one of Inman Park's oldest houses. George E. King, founder of King Hardware Company, had this elegant Victorian house built in 1889. Even though the house was damaged in a fire, its five owners have helped to preserve it. The exterior is painted in Victorian colors.

The 1890 house at number 897 is a good example of the High Victorian–style homes.

Across the street, you will see the Ernest and Emily Winship Woodruff house at number 908. Walter T. Downing, popular architect, designed this twenty-six-room mansion. Robert W. Woodruff, Ernest's son who took over the company from his father, grew up here.

➤Cross Waverly Way.

➤You will pass the 1890 Inman Park Trolley Barn. It remains Atlanta's major artifact of the electric street railway era. Designed in the shingle style characteristic of the High Victorian period in Atlanta, it housed the cars of Hurt's Atlanta and Edgewood Street Railroad Company. Since its restoration, it has been used as a farmers' market, a shoe shop, and a basketball court. It now serves as a community center, and you might even come upon a wedding reception taking place there.

➤Cross Elizabeth Street and come to the end of the walk.

Walk 10
Druid Hills

   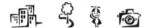

General location: 3 miles northeast of downtown.

Special attractions: Distinctive neighborhood, historic homes, parks, dogwoods in springtime.

Difficulty rating: Easy, with one stretch of hill without a sidewalk.

Distance: 1.3 miles.

Estimated time: 40 minutes.

Services: None.

Restrictions: Dogs must be kept on leashes no longer than 6 feet, and their droppings must be picked up.

For more information: Call Atlanta Convention and Visitors Bureau.

Druid Hills

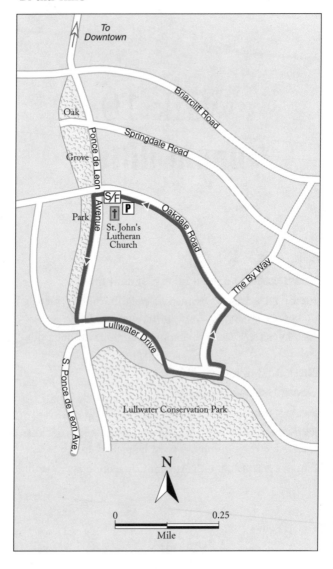

Walk 10

Getting started: From downtown take Peachtree Street north; then turn right on Ponce de Leon Avenue. Turn left on Oakdale Road and park in the church parking lot.

Public transportation: The route number 2 Ponce de Leon MARTA bus runs along Ponce de Leon Avenue. Buses serve the North Avenue and Decatur rapid-rail stations. Call MARTA for current schedules and confirm the bus's destination when you buy the ticket.

Overview: The U.S. Department of the Interior has described the Druid Hills Historic District as "the finest examples of late nineteenth and early twentieth century comprehensive residential planning and development in the Southeast." In turn-of-the-twentieth-century Atlanta, creating new suburban communities became big business. Atlanta developer Joel Hurt hired Frederick Law Olmsted, Jr., commonly known as the father of landscape architecture, in 1892 to design a unique "parkway suburb." Olmsted designed America's first park, New York City's Central Park. He also helped write the Organic Act of 1916, which formed the National Park Service.

He favored a parklike setting for residential neighborhoods; thus he created the 2-mile strip of park bordering Ponce de Leon. Atlanta's leaders had previously had no thought of creating an aesthetic environment. Living in a transportation hub, local people had always hurried.

Olmsted also liked to provide single-family lots where people could live away from the city, yet close to it. He made another unusual suggestion: to locate the electric street railway line on a strip of land adjacent to—rather than in the center of—the roadway. Olmsted died before the completion of Druid Hills, but his sons completed the 1,500-acre project. The gently rolling countryside and the

129

lush greenery enabled this suburb to become one of Olmsted's most beautiful garden suburbs in North America. The first house was built in 1911, and the neighborhood took off by the late 1920s. Presently, many of the city's older neighborhoods reflect the humanizing influence of the meandering roadways, extensive public open space, and landscaped lots of Druid Hills. The district is listed on the National Register of Historic Places.

The Walk

➤The walks starts at St. John's Lutheran Church at 1410 Ponce de Leon Avenue at the corner of Oakdale Road. The church is housed in two buildings—the historic Stonehenge Mansion built in 1914 and the sanctuary, which was added in 1969. Both are built out of Stone Mountain granite. The mansion was built for Samuel Hoyt Venable and his sister and her family. Sam and his brother William owned the Southern Granite Company and Stone Mountain. It was only natural that Sam would choose granite for his home. The church bought the mansion in 1959 and used the same granite when the sanctuary was added.

➤Cross the street and turn left through Oak Grove Park. The park is one of six that Olmsted designed. Plans in the 1950s and 1960s slated the park to be a part of the Freedom Parkway, to connect Stone Mountain with downtown. Partly due to then-Gov. Jimmy Carter's efforts, those plans did not materialize. Some of the trees in the park, such as the Bradford pears, didn't exist in Olmsted's time. The Darlington oak, a variety of live oak, is one of the trees that did exist at that time.

Walk 10

On the right you will pass the Howard School, a private school in a house built for Jacob Elsas, founder of the Fulton Bag and Cotton Mill. You may read about the mill in Walk 4.

Across the street at 1428 Ponce de Leon is the St. John Chrysostom Melkite Catholic Church. The building was originally the private residence of Asa Candler, who founded Coca-Cola.

►Take a left onto Lullwater Drive. This street helps give Atlanta the name Dogwood City. In springtime many streets such as this burst forth into dogwood and azalea blossoms. The Mediterranean-style "Rainbow Villa" at number 761, with a Spanish tile roof, belonged to Lucy Candler Heinz's son and daughter-in-law. Lucy Candler was the only daughter of Asa Candler.

The producers of the film *Driving Miss Daisy* used the Country English Manor–style house at number 822 for filming the movie, in 1989. The producers actually liked the house next door better, but renovations had updated the interior; this one still has its original kitchen. It is a private residence.

►Cross the street and enter the Lullwater Conservation Park, a public park and bird sanctuary built in 1931. Lullwater Creek runs through the park. Mountain laurel and rhododendron—usually found in the North Georgia mountains and seldom found in Atlanta—grow there.

►Cross Lullwater Drive. Asa Candler's grandson built the English Tudor Revival–style house at number 925.

►Turn left and take a right onto The By Way. This short street has no sidewalks but has very little traffic, so you will be safe walking there.

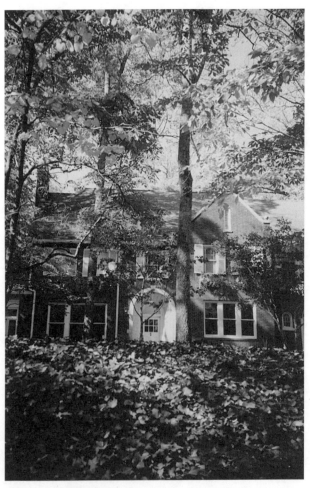

*The Country English Manor–style house at 822 Lullwater Drive
was featured in the 1989 film* Driving Miss Daisy.

Walk 10

During the early days of the neighborhood, servants took streetcars, getting off on Ponce de Leon; they then walked a pathway from Oakdale Road to Lullwater Drive. After being paved, the path received the name The By Way. You will notice some nondescript houses built on this street during the 1960s and 1970s before the raising of awareness about historic preservation. The newer homes obey the requirements from the Historic Preservation Society.

➤Turn left onto Oakdale Road.

Asa Candler Jr. built the house at number 901. He brought wild animals from his foreign travels and put them in his backyard. Because Candler's neighbors objected to his animals, he donated them to the Atlanta Zoo. These included a variety of monkeys and bears, as well as an elephant named Coca.

Louis Elsas, vice president of the Fulton Bag and Cotton Mill in Cabbagetown, lived in the house at number 888.

Popular Atlanta architect Walter T. Downing designed the brick Tudor-style house at number 893 for his family. A later resident operated the first privately owned kindergarten in DeKalb County in the playroom of the house.

Leila Ross Wilburn, a female Atlanta architect who practiced from 1909 until her death in 1967 designed the house at number 871. This house emulates Frank Lloyd Wright's Prairie style. In 1911, Powers Pace, a hardware company executive, built the house at number 858, the first residence in the neighborhood. His daughter, the first baby born in the neighborhood, grew up to become the first young woman to marry there.

Locals call Druid Hills Neil Reed country. A popular Atlanta architect, Neel Reid had studied in Europe. He influenced the quality of Atlanta's best residential areas from the close of World War I to the mid-twenties more than any other architect. He showed his talent most often in houses of Renaissance or Georgian design.

Reid designed the house at number 850 in 1916. The French seventeenth-century château, with Georgian Revival touches, has a massive entrance, typical of Reid's designs. The house belonged to Sigmund Montag, who owned the National Pencil Company and was the uncle of Leo Frank, who was accused of murdering a thirteen-year-old girl at the pencil factory. The grandmother of Alfred Uhry, who wrote *Driving Miss Daisy,* once owned this house. Uhry based the character of Miss Daisy on his grandmother.

Franklin Delano Roosevelt visited the house at number 827 several times on his way to Warm Springs in south Georgia. Charles Sheldon, a prominent attorney who managed FDR's presidential campaign in Georgia, built the house in 1910. He happened to be the only Georgian who signed the Treaty of Versailles.

Al Capone's family rented the house next door at number 835 in 1932, when Capone was in the federal prison in Atlanta. Possibly FDR might have visited next door to the Al Capone family.

Clyde King of the King Plow Company built the house at the corner of Oakdale and Ponce de Leon. Massive Corinthian columns frame the front entrance of this house, which now serves as the national headquarters of the Alpha Delta Pi sorority. A descendant of the Kings said it would please the couple that young people now enjoy the house—a scene of many parties. The back gardens have won many prizes.

➤You have reached the end of the walk.

Walk 11
Midtown

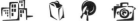

General location: This walk begins 1 mile north of downtown Atlanta.

Special attractions: The Margaret Mitchell House & Museum, Georgia Institute of Technology, Coca-Cola headquarters, the Varsity restaurant, the Fox Theater, old churches, and other historic buildings.

Difficulty rating: Mostly flat, with a couple of inclines; all paved.

Distance: 3.6 miles.

Estimated time: 2 hours.

Services: Restaurants; rest rooms are available at Margaret Mitchell House Visitor Center and Patterson Funeral Home.

Midtown

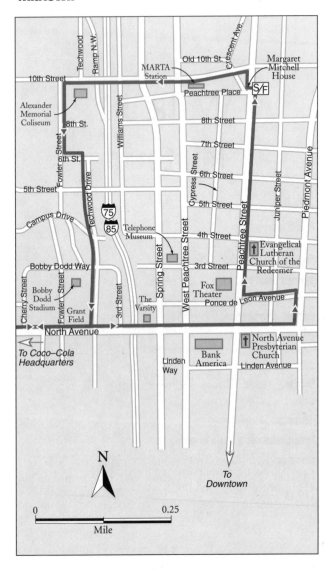

Walk 11

Restrictions: Dogs must be on leashes no longer than 6 feet, and their droppings must be picked up.

For more information: Contact the Atlanta Convention and Visitors Bureau, the Margaret Mitchell House & Museum, World of Coca-Cola Atlanta, and the Georgia Institute of Technology. Call the Atlanta Preservation Center for information about tours of this area March–November.

Getting started: This walk starts at the Margaret Mitchell House & Museum. From I–75 South, take exit 250, and turn left on Tenth Street. Turn right on Peachtree Street, where you will find public parking within the next block. The Mitchell House provides free parking in the lot at Crescent Street only while visiting the house.

Public transportation: Take MARTA bus route number 10 or any northbound train to the midtown MARTA station. Contact MARTA to confirm routes and times, and confirm the bus or train's destination when you buy the ticket.

Overview: After the Civil War locals called the area around Tenth Street "Tight Squeeze," a wooded ravine where the lawless hung out. The narrow road made traveling by wagon difficult. Bandits also hid in the wooded ravine and surrounding forests to rob travelers heading north out of the city. The area became, therefore, a "tight squeeze" for riders trying to pass through with their money and their lives.

During the latter part of the nineteenth century, wealthy people built homes in the area. By the 1900s those homes gave way to office and retail business as the commercial district expanded; and during the 1950s and 1960s, the area housed the South's largest hippie district. But in recent years the area has undergone significant change. In 1999 the Midtown Historic District was listed on the National Register of Historic Places.

The Walk

➤The walk starts at the Margaret Mitchell Visitors Center. The facility houses a small theater and a photo-exhibit gallery of Mitchell during her late teens and early twenties. The Museum Shop has gifts, souvenirs, and *Gone With the Wind* collectibles and memorabilia. Visitors can tour Mitchell's apartment, which is in a mansion across the lawn from the Center, and a movie museum.

Mitchell started writing *Gone With the Wind* during her twenties and worked at it for nine years. She wrote the majority of the book while seated at a typewriter in the small corner alcove of the Peachtree Street apartment. Between 1925 and 1932 Mitchell and her husband, John Marsh, lived in apartment No. 1 on the first floor in the Tudor Revival mansion she affectionately called "The Dump." Their apartment is the only one preserved in the building, and all furnishings come from that the period. The house is one of the two oldest houses still standing on Peachtree Street.

➤After leaving the Margaret Mitchell House, take a left onto Tenth Street. Cross Crescent Avenue and West Peachtree and Spring Streets.

On Spring look on the right for the beautiful white-washed brick mansion, H. M. Patterson Funeral Home. In 1882, when the city still had dirt streets, Patterson started his funeral home downtown. The fifth generation of his family runs the business now. Patterson's welcomes visitors to see the gardens and to use the rest rooms.

Author of the World's Favorite Novel

On November 8, 1900, prominent Atlanta attorney Eugene Mitchell and his wife, Maybelle, welcomed a baby daughter, whom they named Margaret. During the Battle of Atlanta, soldiers had used their house as a hospital. Little Margaret grew up hearing relatives tell stories about the Civil War.

Health problems forced her to become practically bedridden. Her husband would bring bags of books home from the library every evening. He finally told her he thought she could write a book herself. She did, but she kept the project secret from friends and family, throwing a towel over the typewriter when guests came.

A Macmillan editor came to Atlanta in 1935, searching for manuscripts. Mitchell took her work to him, saying, "Take the damn thing before I change my mind." The next day she sent him a telegram, saying, "Send it back; I've changed my mind." The editor had already started reading the manuscript, though. Enthralled, he kept it. The book, *Gone With the Wind,* appeared in 1936, and the movie premiere took place on December 14, 1939, at Atlanta's Loew's Theater.

In 1947 Mitchell received the Pulitzer Prize for literature. For decades her book outsold every other except for the Bible. She never wrote another book.

Mitchell—even though plagued by health problems—spent a lot of time doing volunteer work. She also attended relatives and others when they were sick. She also wrote a letter, by hand, to every fan who wrote to her.

She died on August 16, 1949, at age forty-nine from brain injuries sustained when a drunken taxi driver, Hugh Gravitt, hit her. Her brother carried out her request that her original manuscript be burned after her death. She rests in Historic Oakland Cemetery in the Mitchell family plot. You can read about the cemetery in Walk 5.

➤Cross Williams Street and walk across the bridge over I–75/85. Cross Ramp N.W. You are entering the Georgia Institute of Technology campus.

Sherman's army demolished Atlanta's earliest buildings during the Civil War, and rebuilding proved difficult: People lacked money, materials, skilled craftsmen, engineers, and architects. Most early architects had learned through an apprenticeship system rather than schools; those with formal training had to be imported from the North or from Paris. "The Tech" opened in 1888 to provide the skills necessary to build the New South. The original campus had nine acres and now has 330. Presently Georgia Tech enjoys national renown as a scientific institution.

➤You will pass the Alexander Memorial Coliseum—the "Big Dome"—on the left, home to Tech's outstanding varsity basketball team. Tech calls it the "thriller dome" because of the thrilling wins that have happened there. The renovated building served as the 1996 site for Olympic boxing.

➤Turn left on Fowler Street. You will pass the Bill Moore Tennis Center on the right. Griffin Track Center, called the Rose Bowl Field, lies behind the hedge past the center. Tech's football team won the national championship at the Rose Bowl in California in 1928. That game became famous because of the wrong-way run Roy Reigel—on the opposing team—made. Tech won the game by one point, and the school built the Track Center with the winnings.

➤Cross Eighth Street and turn left on Sixth Street. (*Note:* There is no Seventh Street.)

➤Turn right on Techwood Drive.

➤Cross Fifth Street.

➤Cross Campus Drive.

Walk 11

➤Cross Bobby Dodd Way. You will pass Bobby Dodd Stadium on the right, one of the oldest in use in the United States. Dodd-Grant Field, next to the tower, has been home to Tech's football team since the early 1900s. In the years 1917, 1928, 1952, and 1990, the Yellowjackets won national championships. The most uneven victory in football history took place on this field in 1916 when Tech won over Cumberland College 222–0.

➤At North Avenue turn right and walk uphill. On the right is the original campus. A cluster of mixed-period buildings rests on the crest of the "Hill." The 1888 Administration Building, "Tech Tower," with its Victorian Gothic design, remains the focal point of the campus. Several buildings in this area make up the Georgia Tech Historic District.

➤Cross Fowler and Cherry Streets. The Guggenheim Building for Aerospace Engineering sits on the corner of North and Cherry. Tech's aerospace engineering program is among the top five in the nation.

➤When you reach Tech Parkway, look ahead on the left on North Avenue, to see the Coca-Cola corporate headquarters. You may take a tour of this famous company, whose name is synonymous with Atlanta.

➤Retrace your steps on North, crossing Techwood Drive.

➤Cross the bridge over I–75. As you are walking across, look to the left to see the Centennial Tower beside I–75, built for the 1996 Olympics. The twelve-story green obelisk bears a 16-foot flame at its apex. After you cross I–75 you will pass the Varsity restaurant on the left.

Go to the Varsity, an important Atlanta landmark, for a "cholesterol fix." The world's largest drive-in boasts that it fries everything except Cokes. It serves 350 gallons of

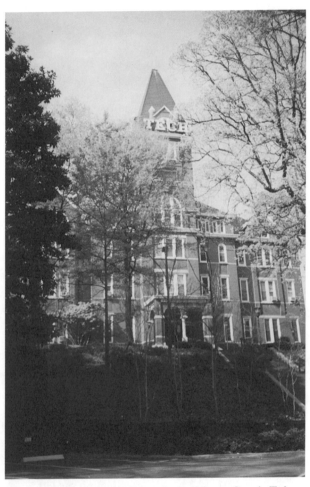

The tower of the 1888 Administration Building at Georgia Tech dominates the campus.

chili and 2 miles of hot dogs every day. The red-shirted servers use their own special language to belt out orders. "F.O. and a naked dog walking" means a frosted orange drink and a plain hot dog to go. Try a chili dog, fried onion rings, chili steak, and a "Varsity Orange" drink.

➤Cross Spring Street.

➤Pass All Saints Episcopal Church at the corner of North and West Peachtree. This 1906 building with red Virginia sandstone walls resembles English parish churches. The seven stained-glass windows came from the Tiffany Studio in New York.

As you look left up West Peachtree, you will see the Southern Bell Telephone Building in its fifty-story granite tower. It houses the Telephone Museum.

➤Cross West Peachtree Street. At 30 North Avenue you will pass Fire Station No. 11, the 1907 structure designed in Italian Renaissance style.

You will be walking beside the BankAmerica Tower, which covers the block between West Peachtree and Peachtree Streets. Its unusual open-framed canopy gives it its nickname as Atlanta's Eiffel Tower. This stone-and-glass skyscraper is the city's tallest building and the ninth tallest in the world. Take a moment to enjoy the flowers and shrubs on its beautiful front lawn.

➤When you reach Peachtree Street, you will see Crawford Long Hospital to the right and 1 block south. The hospital is named for Crawford Williamson Long, a Georgia physician who developed the idea that ether could reduce surgical pain. In 1842 Long painlessly removed a cyst from an anesthetized man in a successful operation using sulphuric ether. He charged $2.00.

➤Cross Peachtree Street. The North Avenue Presbyterian Church is on the right. This 1907 building, with an Old World allure, originally stood among Victorian mansions.

➤Continue walking downhill and cross Juniper Street.

➤Take a left onto Piedmont Avenue. Across the street you will see The Mansion restaurant. One of Atlanta's best preserved old houses, this 1883 Queen Anne house set a trend among the city's middle class and business elite. The house became a restaurant in 1973, and present owners added the gingerbread gazebo on the North Avenue facade.

➤You will pass The Abbey restaurant. Formerly a church built in 1915, it has sixty massive stained-glass windows and a 50-foot arched and vaulted ceiling. The present owners created the atmosphere of a medieval abbey when they opened the restaurant in 1968. They added tapestries, statuary, brass rubbings, monks' chairs, and copperware. Waiters wear hooded monk's garb. The European chefs have earned the restaurant the most awards of any other Atlanta restaurant.

When you reach the corner of Piedmont and Ponce de Leon Avenues—and especially if it is mealtime and you are hungry—you could walk 1 block to the right to Mary Mac's Tea Room. Mary Mac's has been serving sumptuous Southern food since 1945. In early 2001 *Gourmet* magazine named it the best Southern food restaurant in Atlanta. Mary Mac's takes cash only.

➤Take a left onto Ponce de Leon Avenue. Cross Juniper Street and go 1 block to Peachtree Street. On the corner on the left, at number 1913 you will see The Ponce, the first large high-rise luxury apartment building in Atlanta.

➤Cross Peachtree Street and turn right. You will pass the Georgian Terrace across the street, a former hotel that now has apartments. This 1911 Grand Old Lady of Peachtree, one of the great hotels of the Southeast, provided the most luxurious accommodations in Atlanta. Clark Gable and other guests for the world premier of *Gone With the Wind* stayed there in 1939.

You will come to the Fox Theater, the last surviving grand movie palace in Atlanta and America's second-largest movie palace. The theater opened on Christmas Day in 1929. Its exterior resembles a Moorish palace, with lancet arches, minarets, and onion domes. Inside the 4,000-seat auditorium visitors find an Arabian courtyard, where trompe l'oeil stars twinkle in the night sky. The Fox survived the wrecking ball in the 1970s, and volunteers restored it to its original grandeur.

Major theatrical productions and concerts now take place here. In 1989 Ted Turner observed the fiftieth anniversary of *Gone With the Wind* with a special "re-premier" of the cinematically restored film there. Contact the Atlanta Preservation Center about tours.

➤As you continue on Peachtree, you'll see the Days Inn Hotel/Peachtree, which started life in 1925 as the Carlton Bachelor Hotel.

➤At the corner you will pass Agatha's, a dinner theater in an old building. While guests dine, they watch—and participate in—an original mystery comedy production.

➤Cross Third Street. Two old churches are in this area. The Evangelical Lutheran Church of the Redeemer on the right has massive towering walls of rough-hewn, coursed stone in its 1952 building.

➤Cross Fourth Street.

➤Cross Fifth Street. The second old church in this area is Saint Mark United Methodist Church, built in 1903, which resembles a Victorian-era structure. Its Stone Mountain granite ashlar walls are designed in modified Gothic style. Twelve outstanding German pictorial stained-glass windows adorn the building. Notice the carved triple-arched doors.

➤Cross Sixth Street.

➤Cross Eighth Street.

➤When you cross Peachtree Place, turn left and cross Peachtree Street to the end of the walk.

Walk 12

The Atlanta History Center

     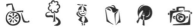

General location: About 6 miles north of downtown.

Special attractions: Trails and gardens, museum, Swan House, Tullie Smith House, farm buildings and animals.

Difficulty rating: Moderate; on dirt trail.

Distance: 0.5 mile.

Estimated time: 15 minutes.

Services: Rest rooms and Coca-Cola Cafe are available in the museum; rest rooms are available in the Coach House Restaurant; there are gift shops in the museum and restaurant. Individuals with physical disabilities can readily access the museum, library/archives, and portions of the gardens. Some of the exhibitions in the museum have large-print

The Atlanta History Center

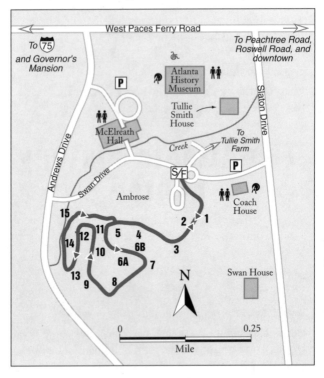

reading materials. Video presentations at the museum have subtitles. Visitors may secure maps in English, French, German, Japanese, and Spanish. Free parking.

Restrictions: The museum, Tullie Smith House, and the Swan House charge admission on a first-come, first-served basis. Ticket sales end at 4:30 p.m.; it takes three hours to tour the museum, houses, and gardens. Ticket prices may change without notice. You may take food and drink only into certain permitted areas. Strollers are permitted outdoors and in the museum but not in the historic houses.

For more information: Call the Atlanta History Center.

Getting started: From downtown on I–75 North, take the West Paces Ferry Road exit 255 and turn left at the end of the ramp onto Northside Parkway. Turn right at the next intersection onto West Paces Ferry Road. Continue east for 2.5 miles to 130 West Paces Ferry. Turn right into Andrews Drive just before the center; then turn left into the parking lot. You may also park on most side streets.

From I–75 South take the West Paces Ferry Road exit and turn left at the end of the ramp onto West Paces Ferry Road. Continue east for 2.5 miles. Follow directions for parking above.

Public transportation: MARTA bus route number 40 runs on West Paces Ferry Road and serves the Lindbergh rapid-rail station. Or take MARTA to the Lenox station or Buckhead/Financial Center station; then take bus number 23 south to Peachtree Road and West Paces Ferry Road. The Atlanta History Center lies 3 blocks west. Call MARTA for current schedules and confirm bus's destination when you buy the ticket.

Overview: Some people call Buckhead "the Beverly Hills of the East." Others call this 28-square-mile area "richnorthwestAtlanta." The first Buckhead residents—prehistoric hunters—lived in the area 7,000 to 8,000 years ago. Indians lived in a village called Standing Peach Tree at the junction of the Chattahoochee River and Peachtree Creek. Under pressure the Indians signed a treaty in 1821,

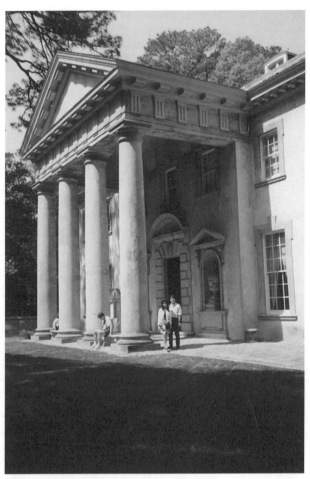

The historic 1928 Swan House draws visitors at the Atlanta History Center.

which gave more than four million acres of their land to Georgia. That area included Standing Peach Tree.

Whites quickly settled the area. Henry Irby cleared land and built a general store, where he sold liquor at the present corner of West Paces Ferry and Roswell Road. In December 1838 Irby shot a large buck at a spring and mounted its head on a post above the store's door. People started referring to the location as "Buck's Head."

Atlanta's growth spurred Buckhead's growth. Farmers passed through there as they brought their produce and livestock south from North Carolina, Tennessee, and Kentucky to Atlanta's markets.

The Civil War touched Buckhead. Between 60,000 to 80,000 Union soldiers forded the Chattahoochee River and entered Buckhead on July 16, 1864. They took shelter in the woods, raided livestock and crops, leaving locals poor and hungry. On July 20, 1864, the Union forces defeated the Confederates at the Battle of Peachtree Creek. The Union troops moved in to Atlanta, fighting the Battle of Atlanta on July 22.

After the Civil War local residents lived in near poverty. Dwellers built gristmills, sawmills and pottery factories. Buckhead had a large quantity of quality clay, and during the late 1870s and 1880s, it became one of the state's eight main pottery-making centers.

In 1866 people discovered gold on Nancy Creek in the area, and a man named Henry Irby started prospecting. At the end of the war, he owned lots of land, but he had only worthless Confederate currency. He bartered away some of his land for 5 cents an acre to buy needed goods, such as exchanging land for wheat. Irby died in February 1879.

Atlanta History Center

This stop provides delights for all the senses: sights, sounds, touch, taste, and smells. You will find yourself inside thirty-three acres of beautiful gardens, woodlands, and nature trails that reflect the horticultural history of the Atlanta region.

The museum has three permanent exhibits as well as temporary exhibits. It features the fifth-largest Civil War display in the nation, Southern folk arts, and the Bobby Jones exhibit, which gives a history of golf.

After leaving the exhibit areas, go downstairs to the Coca-Cola Cafe to drink a chocolate Coke, an Atlanta thing.

You may want to tour the majestic 1928 Italianate palazzo Swan House, built by Philip Trammell Shutze, one of the twentieth century's greatest classical architects. Edward Inman, heir to a cotton brokerage fortune, and his wife, Emily, lived there. The house shows the lifestyle of the wealthy in 1930s Atlanta and contains original furnishings. A grand spiral staircase rises from a marble floor. It also houses the Philip Trammell Shutze Collection of Decorative Arts. The house stands on twenty-eight acres of expansive grounds, with lush formal gardens and terraced lawns.

You would enjoy eating lunch at the elegant Swan Coach House Restaurant. The building first served as the garage and servants' quarters of the Swan House. It features uniquely decorated rooms, a fine-arts gallery, and a canopied terrace overlooking a formal garden.

While there, visit the Tullie Smith house, one of the oldest standing houses in the Atlanta area and one of the few that survived the Civil War. It offers a taste of rural life in Piedmont Georgia before the Civil War, complete with a farmhouse, kitchen, barn, and outbuildings. Yeoman farmer Robert Smith built the house in the 1840s near Atlanta, and the center moved it here. A yeoman farmer worked alongside his slaves—in contrast to a plantation owner, who did not. Smith's descendants lived in the house until 1967. Inside you will see plantation-made furniture and historic Staffordshire on display. Docents demonstrate nineteenth-century crafts, such as spinning and open-hearth cooking. A period garden surrounds the property.

The center's gardens provide a horticultural history of Atlanta, starting with the landscape at the front of the museum, which depicts the evolution of a Piedmont forest. You can see an Asian-American garden, a rhododendron garden, and a garden of native plants.

In 1900 the most famous landmark, his log tavern, came down.

In the early 1900s Atlanta residents escaped the heat of downtown into summer cottages they built in Buckhead "in the country."

The state Prohibition in 1907 initiated the demise of Georgia's folk-pottery tradition. The Depression, mass production of metal and glass containers, and the rise of commercial dairies—which reduced the demand for equipment used in home processing—finished it.

In 1952 Atlanta annexed Buckhead, and the area now has one of the most beautiful residential sections in the nation. The governor of Georgia also lives there.

The Walk

Swan Woods Trail

➤Start at the entrance to the trail on Swan Drive beside the driveway to the Swan House. This ten-acre woodland was developed as an outdoor laboratory in the 1970s. The forest has two distinctly different areas. The upper part is a mature virgin forest of oak, hickory, and pine. The lower slope, a former cotton field, has an understory of shrubs and hardwoods, with an advanced secondary growth of pines. Follow the numbered stations along the way that explain what you will see.

The first station stops at the overlook. You have a view into the interior of a forest typical of the great deciduous (leaf-shedding) forests of the Southern Appalachian Mountains and Upper Piedmont Plateau. The canopy includes tulip poplar, American beech, and several kinds of oak and hickory.

The second station tells about the amazing variety of warm-blooded animals found here, surprising for woods located in a metropolitan area.

The third station speaks of the checks and balances that enable an ecosystem to maintain itself. For example, usually a foreign organism fails to survive when introduced into a natural system. Within this forest you see exceptions to that rule, however: English ivy, bamboo, and Japanese honeysuckle. The system had not developed the necessary controls to keep the system within balance.

As you walk downhill, look for a sprinkling of evergreen magnolias. On the right you will see the Swan House boxwood gardens and the magnolias that surround them.

When you reach the fourth station, you have reached the beginning of the cotton field. Some of the terraces and erosion gullies still remain from the 1920s when cotton last grew here. About eighty years ago the farmer abandoned this field. Within five years annual and perennial plants invaded the field, making the establishment of pine trees possible. Hardwoods grew under the dense shade of the pine canopy within the next five years, leading to the death of the pines.

Look to the right to see Ambrose, the marble elephant who resides on the Swan House grounds. Ambrose was "born" in 1894, weighing around 18,700 pounds. It took two wagons and eight horses to move him in front of the White Elephant Saloon, where he stood for twenty years. The Atlanta Historical Society brought him back here in 1971.

As you walk down the hill to the fifth station, you will see the Fern Circle, a part of the original Swan House landscape, against a background of rhododendrons. Native trillium and wild ginger border the circle.

►Bear left.

A magnificent stand of dogwoods greets you at the 6A station.

Station 6B shows how a forest is a mosaic of communities, brought about in part by gaps caused by natural and human events. Two separate tornadoes that blew over tall trees and invasions by the southern pine beetle have opened up this area several times.

The semiopen areas in the 7A station permit sunlight to enter, and you will see plants that bloom and bear fruit. These plants provide the principal sources of food for birds.

As you walk downhill to station 8, you will see the mature eighty-year-old pines that have fallen prey to storm and insect damage. This loss, which always comes to mature and overage trees, releases the understory hardwoods from competition for light, moisture, and food and thus accelerates restoration of the original hardwood forest. You will see meadow flowers and shrubs in the open areas.

As you continue downhill to station 9A, you will see fungi, algae, lichens, mosses, and ferns if you have a sharp eye.

This area is home to a representative collection of native North Georgia magnolia species that bloom in the spring. The big-leaf magnolia has the largest leaf of any deciduous tree in the United States, with some leaves growing a yard long. The umbrella magnolia has leaves that can grow 2 feet long.

As you reach station 10, take a look at the forest floor. Beneath it a great part of the forest lies unseen, where decomposition of dead plants and animals takes place to continue one of the great cycles of life.

As you reach station 11, you will see examples of various kinds of native azaleas found in Georgia that bloom from spring through August.

As you pass station 12, the path winds through the bottom land bounded by hillside and stream. Along its edges you will find a wide range of natural woodland flowers that bloom in the spring.

You will then come to the Garden for Peace.

Station 13 explains food chains and webs essential to our existence.

Station 14 speaks of the various-size animals that play a part in the ecosystem. By far the most numerous animals

Walk 12

Of Interest

Garden for Peace

Atlanta physician Laura Dorsey got an idea for creating a garden network when she went to Japan to care for her husband, who had been wounded in the Vietnam War. Spending time in Japanese gardens helped her handle the stress and rigors of a military hospital.

Over the years Dr. Dorsey realized that the feelings people get from gardens transcend world conflict. She also saw that time spent in gardens provides moments for personal reflection, meditation, and renewal. In 1984 she organized a nonprofit organization, Gardens for Peace, that works to make others more aware of the significance of the garden as a peace symbol. It also encourages individuals and nations to seek peaceful solutions thorough dialogue.

In 1988 the organization dedicated its first garden here. It had a sculptural exchange with one of Atlanta's Sister Cities, Tbilisi, Georgia, in what was then the Soviet Union. Georgian artist Georgia "Gia" Japaridze sculpted *The Peace Tree,* a life-size bronze that stands here.

are the insects. Some of the less frequent animals are the cold-blooded vertebrates such as snakes, turtles, frogs, and fish, while others are microscopic.

Station 15 points out the permanent stream that arises from a small watershed of only a few acres and flows throughout the year.

►Continue uphill on the trail. At station 5, you begin to retrace your steps to the beginning of the walk.

The Governor's Mansion

The governor's mansion, called the State Executive Center, stands on eighteen acres at 391 West Paces Ferry Road, 1 mile northwest of the Atlanta History Museum.

The Georgia General Assembly Committee specified that they wanted a "new mansion that should be in keeping with Georgia's Southern heritage." The neo-Palladian architectural character of the thirty-room mansion shows the influence of the Jeffersonian Classical Revival. The unusually large scale makes it more like the Classical Revival of the Gulf Coast than that of Georgia.

Thirty fluted Doric columns made of California redwood surround the house, making it one of the largest columned houses ever built in the South. The $2-million mansion, completed in 1966, serves as a family residence and as a venue for state occasions. A fine-arts committee assembled a nationally recognized collection of early nineteenth-century antiques and art objects as furnishings. The American furniture constitutes one of the finest collections of Federal-period furniture in the United States.

The west side of the mansion has a sunken, terraced garden.

Walk 13

Atlanta University Center

General location: This unique center for higher education lies 1 mile west of downtown.

Special attractions: The largest consortium of black colleges in the world, including Morehouse College, the alma mater of Martin Luther King Jr.

Difficulty rating: Easy; all on sidewalks. All campuses except that of Morris Brown College, which rests on one of Atlanta's highest points, lie on level ground; all paved.

Distance: 3 miles.

Estimated time: 1.5 hours.

Atlanta University Center

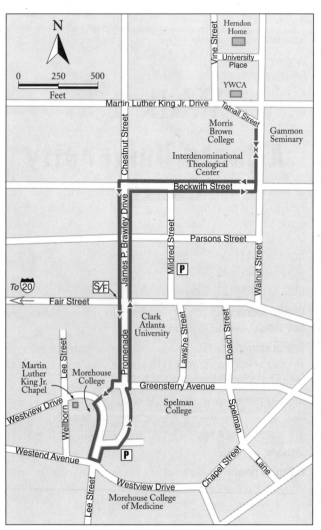

Walk 13

Services: Rest rooms are available in administration and classroom buildings; fast-food places are located on Ashby Street near I–20.

Restrictions: Dogs must be on a leash no longer than 6 feet, and their droppings must be picked up.

For more information: Call the Atlanta Convention and Visitors Bureau.

Getting started: This walk begins at the corner of Fair Street and James P. Brawley Drive. To reach the campus from downtown Atlanta, take I–10 to Ashby Street exit 55A, turn right, and go 0.5 mile to Fair Street. Go 0.2 mile and go through the light at James P. Brawley Drive. Turn left at Mildred Street and park on the deck. It will be hard to find parking on campus during school sessions. On weekends and during summer, you will find ample parking along campus streets, especially on Beckwith and Fair Streets and James P. Brawley Drive.

Public transportation: Take MARTA bus route number 13. Call MARTA for current schedules and confirm the bus's destination when you buy the ticket.

Overview: You will stroll rolling, tree-shaded hills as you tour the Atlanta University campus, which is listed on the National Register of Historic Places. The area has a rich historical background.

By law, slaves could neither read nor write before or during the Civil War. In 1865 Atlanta lay smoldering in ruins from the devastating fires of the Civil War. With the emancipation of the slaves, thousands of destitute former slaves flocked to Atlanta. White missionaries and philanthropists from the North made black education a priority and did missionary work among this population. Blacks had already begun to form schools, but the instructors had little education themselves.

Two ministers ran three grammar schools in 1865 that grew into Atlanta University. In 1867 nine white and two black men applied for a twenty-year charter. Atlanta University began operations on land now occupied by Morris Brown College, at first teaching students of all ages. Children came during the day and adults at night.

Atlanta University (AU) is now the graduate school of the six-institution consortium. Over the years the colleges united, sharing faculty, facilities, and programs. The Morehouse College of Medicine, founded in 1975, became the sixth member of the Atlanta University complex in 1982. At present the institutions the original missionaries and philanthropists helped found form the largest center for black education in the world.

The Walk

➤Start at the gated entrance to Clark Atlanta University. *Essence* magazine, February 1998, listed it among the top five "Best Black College Buys." Follow the beautifully paved Promenade. You will pass Harkness Hall, the CAU administration building. Its gold-topped dome copies the one on the state capitol; however, its gold comes from paint.

On the left you will see buildings with the name Clark College on them. Methodist Episcopal Church leaders started Clark in 1868 in one room of a church to train "good scholars and good teachers." Clark also trained harness makers and wood and iron workers. It now has strong programs in education and the arts. Spike Lee, movie director, graduated from Morehouse but learned cinematography at Clark.

On the right are the buildings of former Atlanta University. The two colleges now make up Clark Atlanta University. The university houses one of the nation's best Afro-American art collections in the Trevor-Arnett Building, the last building on the right. You may want to walk up to the quadrangle to see the sculpture *Spiritual Time* on the upper end of the quadrangle. Artist Frank Toby Martin completed the work for the 1996 Olympics.

The school's $33-million Dolphus E. Milligan Science Research Center on the far side of Trevor-Arnett came about through a collaboration with federal, state, local, and private industries. This is one of the largest university research facilities in the Southeast. Undergraduate students take classes here, whereas in most schools, only graduate students take part in research projects. The university's Mass Communications Department, which has its own radio station, rates number 1 in the Southeast and is among the top three in the nation.

►At the end of the Promenade, walk through the gates. You will be facing Spelman College. Two white female Massachusetts Baptist missionaries founded it in 1881, responding to a seed gift of $100 and a letter from former slaves. They formed the oldest college for black women in the country, and the first classes met in the basement of a church. In 1883 the founders bought some post–Civil War U.S. Army barracks in West Atlanta, which became the present campus. Beginning in the 1880s John D. Rockefeller Sr., gave generously to the school, and his family has continued that practice. The college received its present name in 1884 from Rockefeller's mother-in-law, Lucy Henry Spelman.

Spelman is regarded as the best place in the country for African-Americans to attend college. The Flemish bond brickwork pattern of many buildings distinguishes them from the surrounding campuses. This campus has the most and the oldest magnolia trees—some more than one hundred years old—of any other in the university. You would enjoy strolling around the quadrangle, with buildings around the green, modeled after New England colleges.

The beautiful modern building straight ahead will surely catch your eye. Comedian Bill Cosby and his wife gave $20 million for the Cosby Academic Center completed in 1996.

➤Turn right on Greensferry Avenue; where it curves left, walk straight downhill on the sidewalk. Cross Westview Drive to Morehouse College. Morehouse began in Augusta, Georgia, in 1867 to prepare black men for the ministry and teaching. The present fifty-five-acre campus encompasses a Civil War historic site where Confederate soldiers staged a stubborn resistance during the 1864 Siege of Atlanta. The school now offers a four-year liberal arts program for men. It enjoys an international reputation for producing leaders who have influenced national and world history. The 1889 Graves Hall dominates the campus, the first building erected on the original fourteen acres of this site.

Downhill, to the right, you will see the Martin Luther King Jr. International Chapel and the large statue of King in front. Both King and his father graduated from the school. Spike Lee is another famous graduate.

➤Turn left and walk to the corner of Westend Drive.

➤Turn left and cross Westview. Look across the street to the right to see the Morehouse College of Medicine.

Walk 13

➤Turn left and turn right on the driveway that leads into the Spelman parking lot, which proves that parking lots don't have to be ugly. Turn left and walk uphill and bear right. Cross the street in front of Spelman. Retrace your steps down the Promenade and return to the starting point.

➤Cross Fair Street and walk down the Promenade.

➤Cross Parsons Street. You will pass the 1982 Robert W. Woodruff Library, which houses one of the largest archival collections of black literature in the world. It serves the six colleges on the campus.

➤Turn right on Beckwith Street. CAU spills over onto the surrounding blocks.

On the left you will pass the Interdenominational Theological Center (ITC), which has six individual denominational seminaries. Take the time to walk around its tranquil quadrangle.

Before the Civil War, slaves had attended their masters' churches; then after the war, they started establishing their own churches. That led to the need to educate their own ministers, and the ITC came into being in 1958. More than 35 percent of all trained black ministers in the world and more than 50 percent of all black military chaplains have graduated from ITC.

You will pass Gammon Theological Seminary, established in 1883.

➤Turn left on Walnut Street. You will see an addition to Gammon on the right. Walk 1 block to Morris Brown College and its peaceful campus. The school, the smallest of the AU colleges, calls itself the gateway to downtown Atlanta.

Atlanta University began operations here in 1869. Morris Brown College, Atlanta's oldest institution of higher learning, is the only AU school founded by blacks. It started in the basement of Big Bethel AME Church, Atlanta's oldest African-American church. You will see that church on Walk 3, the Sweet Auburn/Martin Luther King, Jr. District.

The Romanesque Revival Fountain Hall dominates the campus. This building is one of the few surviving buildings designed by Swedish-born architect Gottfried L. Norrman, who practiced in Atlanta from 1880 until his death in 1909. From the third floor you can look out over the city.

Directly in front of the building you will see the gravesite of the first AU president, Edmund Asa Ware. Ware, white, steadfastly opposed the segregation of the races and did not want to be buried in the "whites only" section of the cemetery. Since the conventions of the time forbade his family to bury him in the "colored" section, the school buried him in 1885 in the middle of the road that separated the two sections of the cemetery. In 1894 the university moved his body to the campus. Students brought a 17,000-pound granite boulder from Ware's Massachusetts birthplace to place over his grave.

The 1869 Gaines Hall, the oldest university building in Atlanta, across the bridge, is the second-oldest public building in Atlanta.

Look across the street to see the Phyllis Wheatly Branch of the YWCA. This historic branch was originally founded in 1919 on the east side of town. The present 1950 facility came about as a result of the first and longest building campaign in the history of the Atlanta "Y."

►You may want to turn left on Tatnall Street, cross Martin Luther King Jr. Drive to Vine Street and then turn right on University Place. Walk downhill to the 1910

Alonzo F. Herndon Home museum on the left, which has a commanding view of downtown Atlanta. Herndon— millionaire black businessman—built this home. His wife, Adrienne, an Atlanta University professor and a Shake-spearean actress, decorated it.

►Retrace your steps and return to the beginning of the walk.

Walk 14

Outdoor Activity Center

General location: 2.5 miles from downtown.

Special attractions: Walking trail in hardwood forest; natural science museum; composting demonstration site.

Difficulty rating: Moderate, with uphill.

Distance: 0.75 mile.

Estimated time: 25 minutes.

Services: Rest rooms, water fountains, free parking, playground, and picnic tables are available. Running and jogging are permitted on the trails. Ask about other trails.

Restrictions: There is a $4.00-per-person charge for guided hikes and special activities; self-guided tours are free. Walk only on the paved trail. No smoking allowed. Children

Outdoor Activity Center

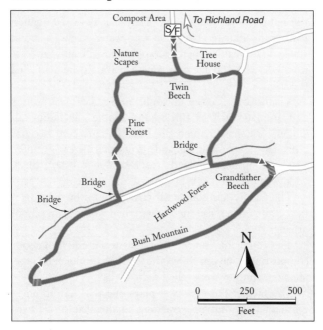

twelve years of age and under must be accompanied by adults or must visit the forest in supervised groups. Do not disturb any snakes or other animals you might see. Take nothing from the forest. Watch out for poison ivy on the trail; ask someone in the center to identify it for you if needed.

For more information: Call Outdoor Activity Center.

Overview: The center, Atlanta's forest in the city, sits on twenty-six heavily forested acres and has 3 ½ miles of hiking trails. The center has operated for the past twenty-five years. Before visitors tour the grounds, they walk through the natural science museum. They can see a 700-gallon fish tank that resembles a freshwater Georgia pond stocked with catfish, perch, crappie, bluegill, and gar. Visitors who come at feeding time can watch the staff feed the fish.

Visitors can also see an exhibit of Smokey Bear posters and animals such as turtles and reptiles, including an albino corn snake named Big Red. The museum also has a display case of animals and plants that dwell in inner-city buildings; they include roaches, a centipede, a black widow spider, an English sparrow, and a pigeon.

The facility has a huge activity room for birthday parties. Children can use the library when working on school projects.

The center has several bins that teach children about composting. One bin shows the finished product and contains fat, slimy worms called red wigglers.

The facility boasts a cool playscape that has an environmental theme with structures in the shapes of leaves and flower petals. Another structure has a burrow and a cave, and a slide that resembles a waterfall. Families can use the ropes course for a team-building exercise, and a tree house has a surrounding deck.

A special program, Science Beyond the Classroom, brings 12,000–15,000 seventh-grade children to the center every year.

One of the popular trees is a huge beech that the staff has dubbed Twin Beech, because it looks like two trees with one trunk. Although it's against the rules, visitors have carved on it. Someone called "Dirty Red," for example, left his or her inscription on it in 1988.

Walk 14

The trail is just long enough to enjoy with small children without having to carry them back to the museum.

Getting started: Take exit 55A off I–20 onto Ashby Street. Turn left at the bottom of the ramp. Drive 0.2 mile and turn right on Ralph W. Abernathy Boulevard; after 0.9 mile it becomes Cascade Street. Drive 0.3 mile and turn left onto Beecher Street; then go 0.15 mile to Rochelle Street. Turn left and go 0.1 mile to a dead end. Turn right onto Richland Street. You will find the center 0.1 mile on the left.

Public transportation: Take the MARTA train to the West End station. Take the number 71 bus to the Beecher Street stop. You would have a five-minute walk to the center. Call MARTA for current bus number and schedules and confirm the bus's destination when you buy the ticket.

The Walk

►The trail starts as you exit the museum. Pass the playscape on the right and bear left. Look on the right to see a twin beech tree. As you walk downhill, the trail turns to the right across a meadow. Follow the path marked by tree limbs laid on the ground.

►Bear left and walk across the bridge as you enter the hardwood forest.

►Bear left. Look for English ivy, heartleaves, and ferns as you walk. Flaming azaleas, which are on the state's endangered list, bloom here in spring.

►You are entering a beech forest. Beeches, which are deciduous hardwoods, grow up to 100 feet in height and up to 3 feet in diameter. The smooth bark, one of the tree's

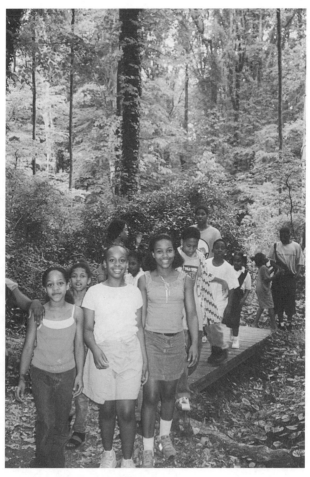

Youngsters from an after-school program enjoy hiking on the trail.

distinctive features, turns out to invite people to carve their initials into it, although it's against the rules.

➤You will reach the Grandfather Beech, a 150-year-old tree—its age measured by girth—so called because it has sworls revealing eyes, nose, and a mouth.

➤Turn right up the steps. You are now on Bush Mountain, 1,052 feet above sea level, the highest elevation on this side of town. The mountain may have gotten its name from bushes that grew there years ago. One of Atlanta's first communities of color, called the Bush community, is at the top of the mountain.

Listen for birds—such as robins, titmice, blue jays, wrens, and pileated woodpeckers—as you walk.

➤Bear right at the trail's fork.

➤As you walk down some steps, you will see a dry streambed on the left.

➤When you reach the bottom of the mountain, pass the bridge and bear right.

➤Cross the second bridge, turn left, and bear right at the dead end.

➤Climb the hill through a pine forest.

➤Turn right at the top of the hill and go through the gate to the end of the walk.

Walk 15

Fernbank Science Center and Museum of Natural History

  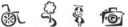

General location: About 8 miles from downtown.

Special attractions: Walking trail in hardwood forest, exhibit hall, planetarium, greenhouse and gardens, composting demonstration site.

Difficulty rating: Moderate with uphill stretch; all paved.

Distance: 0.8 mile.

Estimated time: 25 minutes.

Services: Rest rooms and water fountains are available; an Easy Effort Trail is marked for persons with physical impairments.

Fernbank Science Center and Museum of Natural History

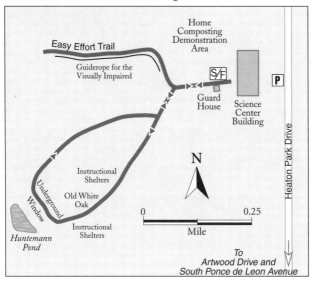

Restrictions: Museum charges admission. Walk only on the paved trail. Smoking, dogs, picnicking, running, jogging, bicycles, or motorized vehicles are not allowed. Children twelve years of age and under must be accompanied by adults or must visit the forest in supervised groups. Do not disturb any snakes or other animals you might see. Take nothing from the forest.

For more information: Call Fernbank Museum of Natural History or Fernbank Science Center.

Getting started: This walk begins at Fernbank Forest behind Fernbank Science Center. Turn off Ponce de Leon Avenue onto Artwood Drive and turn right after 0.2 mile on Heaton Park Drive. The center is on the left.

To reach the Fernbank Museum of Natural History, which is 0.7 mile away, retrace your steps to Ponce de Leon Avenue and turn right. Turn right on Clifton Road; then turn right into the museum area.

Public transportation: Take the number 2 Ponce de Leon MARTA bus to Artwood Drive. Walk up the hill $1\frac{1}{2}$ blocks. Call MARTA for current schedules and confirm the bus's destination when you buy the ticket.

Overview: Fernbank Forest is a sixty-five-acre natural area owned by Fernbank, Inc. and leased to the DeKalb County School System for use as a "living laboratory." During school hours Fernbank instructors teach students. The center is open to the public also.

The family that owned the propperty around 1900 found an abundance of ferns and fern relatives growing in this primeval woodland. They therefore chose the name Fernbank Forest.

The forest has more than thirty species of trees as well as many shrubs and vines. About half of the evergreen plants that you see are introduced plants; that is, they did not originate here but came from another part of the South or even from another part of the world. Others are native plants that have been growing here for thousands of years.

Look for small animals, such as squirrels, and listen for songbirds in the trees.

The leaves do not change color here until the first of November. Then, for two or three weeks, the landscape is ablaze with a beauty that can be seen nowhere except in the eastern United States, in western Europe, and in southeastern Asia. The sufficient variety of deciduous trees that causes the beautiful change in scenery takes place only in these parts of the world.

The Walk

➤Start the walk at the gate. On the left look at the sweet-gum trees leaning over the trail. Strong winds accompanying a mid-afternoon storm during the summer of 1986 blew these trees almost to the ground. Sweet-gum wood is tough and fibrous, so the trees did not snap but bent. As the years pass they will continue to grow toward the forest canopy, but they will never be as straight as they were before the storm.

The trail to the right is the Easy Effort trail. Go about 0.5 mile to the point where the trail turns to the left and retrace the path.

➤Follow the trail to the left. Notice a fallen tree on the right and look for others as you walk along. On October 5, 1995, the winds of Hurricane Opal came through the Atlanta area, knocking down trees and power lines. In this forest winds blew down or damaged more than 300 trees. If you look up when standing near a fallen tree, you will probably see the sky. Because Fernbank is an old-growth hardwood forest, it has a closed canopy, but when a large tree falls, it creates an opening in the canopy. Sunlight can then reach the ground, and smaller trees can use the sunlight energy to grow faster.

You will see poison ivy along the trail, especially on the left just before you reach the trail that comes in from the right. Since the forest is managed as a natural area, native plants are allowed to grow as part of the forest ecosystem. Although poison ivy may cause many people to have a skin rash, it provides food and shelter for some of the forest inhabitants. Workers trim it only when it begins to over-grow the trail. Be careful not to touch it.

You will notice only large pines here. Young pines need lots of sunshine to grow well. Many hardwoods, however, can grow well in shade. For the last one hundred years, hardwoods have been dominating the forest, causing the large pines to gradually die out. Since pine seeds do not germinate and grow well in shade, few new pines are growing.

➤Look on the right across from a large northern red oak tree that has been cut on the left. A picnic shelter stood on this spot prior to 1966. Picnickers compacted the soil and prevented the growth of many native plants. Much time must pass before a fragile natural area recovers from human damage such as this.

➤As you go down the hill, look on the right across from some logs on the left, where you will see a concentration of native plants. In 1996, when a large lake was flooding an area of native plants in South Carolina, Fernbank staff members rescued some of the threatened plants and trans-planted them here, where they flourished. Look for OCONEE BELL signs; this plant is extremely rare, found only in a few areas in the mountains of Georgia and the Carolinas.

➤Look to the left to see a few small magnolia trees with large evergreen leaves. These trees are not native to the Georgia Piedmont. The scattered trees growing here are "volunteers" that sprouted from seeds brought by animals from trees planted in residential areas.

You will see many dead pines in the forest. The south-ern pine beetle killed more than one third of the pines here in the early 1970s. Many of the dead trees eventually fell to the ground. Those closest to the trail were cut to prevent possible harm to visitors. More than twenty years later you can see the remains of these once magnificent trees.

►Look at the large white oak tree with the number 5 sign at its base. Perhaps 200 years old, it grew taller than its neighbors and has been lucky to escape lightning, wind damage, ice storms, disease—and the woodsman's ax.

►At the bottom of the hill, you now come to Huntemann Pond, first constructed around 1900. The present pond, built in 1966, is home to an abundance of aquatic life.

Of Interest

The Robert L. Staton Rose Garden

The Fernbank Museum of Natural History's beautiful grounds feature the Robert L. Staton Rose Garden. This garden, open daily to the public free of charge, is located near downtown Atlanta at 767 Clifton Road. It is one of only three gardens in the United States that have both All American Rose Selections (AARS) and American Rose Society (ARS) test roses.

The garden bears the name of the man who first established a rose garden at Fernbank in 1983. Bob Staton developed a love of roses as a child and joined the American Rose Society as a teenager. He later became a trained horticulturist and worked at the museum. His desire to educate the public and the absence of a test site in Atlanta's growing climate led him to develop the garden.

The garden has approximately 1,300 roses from three sources: All American Rose Selections (AARS) test plants, American Rose Society Award of Excellence Miniature (ARS) test plants, and donated named roses.

At the garden you will see some of Bob's favorite roses, such as 'Garden Party,' 'Tropicana,' 'Double Delight,' and 'Olympiad.'

Look to the left to see rosebay rhododendrons on the bank above the pond. These plants are natives of the North Georgia mountains and were planted here in the winter of 1967.

➤You will pass the closed underground window with a plate glass behind the wooden doors. The doors open only during outdoor classes to allow students to see a profile of the forest soil, roots of trees, worms, and the like. If the doors were left open, conditions would change drastically. Umbrella magnolias, native to this forest, and southern magnolias grow side by side here.

➤Turn right uphill past the underground window.

Look for beech trees where people have carved initials in the bark. You can help protect this beautiful woodland by leaving it exactly as you found it.

If you walk here in spring, look for blooming redbuds and dogwoods farther up the hill on the left.

➤Turn left at the dead end and return to the end of the walk.

As you leave the forest, walk through the Home Composting Demonstration Garden.

Look at the native and ornamental species that have been planted in this area.

Walk 16
Stone Mountain Park

    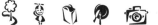

General location: You will find a popular spot for hiking and other recreations in this 3,200-acre park 16 miles east of downtown Atlanta.

Special attractions: Stone Mountain, a skylift, swimming and boating, a steam-train ride, hiking, a nature trail, museums, a petting zoo, golf, and a laser show.

Difficulty rating: Easy; uphill, with places to rest; dirt trail.

Distance: 0.75 mile.

Estimated time: 20 minutes.

Services: Restaurants, rest rooms at information center, gift shop. You can get detailed trail maps and directions at the park information desks.

Stone Mountain Park

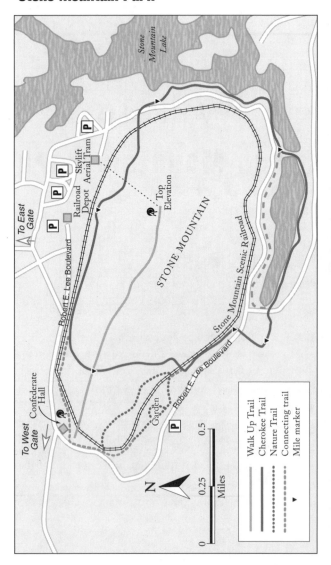

Walk 16

Restrictions: The gates open every day year-round, from 6:00 A.M. to midnight. Major attractions open at 10:00 A.M.; however, due to weather conditions and seasonal schedules, closing times vary. Call for attraction information. Dogs must be on leashes no longer than 6 feet, and their droppings must be picked up.

For more information: Call Stone Mountain Memorial Park.

Getting started: Take I–285 to Stone Mountain Parkway 78, exit 30; then drive east about 5 miles to the park entrance. From downtown, take Ponce de Leon Avenue east; then follow Scott Boulevard, which becomes Lawrenceville Highway. Bear right onto Stone Mountain Parkway to the park entrance. The park has several parking lots.

Public transportation: MARTA buses run regularly. Take route number 120 Stone Mountain, which runs between the Avondale station and Stone Mountain Village just west of the park entrance.

Overview: The state's most popular recreation destination, this park offers many enjoyable activities for children. Stone Mountain won first place in an *Atlanta Journal-Constitution* survey for best place for a day hike, for a picnic, and to take out-of-town visitors. As the owners say, you can have "rock solid fun!"

Two-hundred-million-year-old Stone Mountain, the largest outcropping of exposed granite in the world, rises 800 feet above the surrounding plain. Geologists call this mound of rock a "monadnock" and say it is older than the Pyrenees, the Rockies, or the Himalayas. They believe that 300 million years of erosion uncovered the portion that we now see. The bald dome is home to some rare plants and trees that grow in no other place. Some of these trees may be 800 years old. A former mayor of Atlanta said it was the

Stone Mountain Park Nature Trail

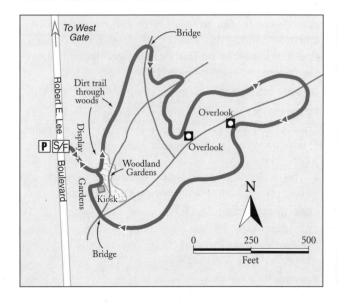

only thing about Atlanta that Sherman didn't burn or the Yankee carpetbaggers cart away.

Humans first came to the mountain between 8,000 and 10,000 years ago, drawn by the game and water supplies. Early Native Americans used it for religious and ceremonial purposes. Modern Native Americans met at the mountain, and early settlers used it as a signpost. Spanish explorers coming from Florida in the late 1500s probably were the first Europeans to see it.

By 1839 trains ran to Stone Mountain, enabling a town to develop. Prior to the Civil War, the area had a reputation as "Atlanta's favorite picnic ground" and as a summer resort.

Walk 16

The Venable brothers, Sam and William, bought Stone Mountain in 1887 for $48,000. Welshmen and Scotchmen quarried there for years. Stone Mountain has been called "the largest deposit of merchantable granite in the world." Millions of tons of its granite have built Atlanta institutions and hundreds of post offices all over the United States and in Cuba.

The state bought the mountain—which Georgians have always called the eighth wonder of the world—in 1959 for $1 million-plus.

On the northern face of the mountain, a perpendicular cliff nearly fifty stories tall, you will see a carving of Confederate generals Robert E. Lee and Stonewall Jackson and Confederate Pres. Jefferson Davis, the world's largest piece of sculpture. After the sculpture's completion in 1970, the theme park opened. Developers scoured the state to assemble everything that might interest visitors to the South. They built a 5-mile scenic railroad, dams, and a lake. The park now draws millions of visitors a year. Only the Disney theme parks in Orlando, Florida, attract more people.

More recently, nature lovers have flocked there to enjoy the incredible natural beauty that surrounds the mountain. Dogwood and flowers bloom in spring and summer, and, in fall, the leaves on the dense hardwoods make a spectacular scene. The park has some small, enchanting, out of-the-way nooks and crannies, lovely places to pause or rest. It is traditional to picnic at Stone Mountain.

The Scenic Railroad makes a 5-mile trip around the base of the mountain, a great treat for kids. The little train, *General II,* gets its name from the one made famous in the Great Locomotive Chase during the Civil War. Along the route passengers pass by two villages: one patterned after a pioneer North Georgia settlement and the other a make-believe Indian village.

Visitors may take the skylift in a cable car to the mountaintop to see one of the area's most beautiful views.

The sound-and-light laser show features high-tech fireworks accompanied by music. The show beams on the side of the mountain while guests sit on the grass.

The 732-bell Carillon provides daily concerts. The Carillon was donated to the park after being exhibited in the 1964 World's Fair.

The nationally ranked golf course stays open seven days a week. Facilities include a 36-hole course, a practice green, a driving range, and a new clubhouse, which features a restaurant, a complete pro shop, a lounge, and banquet facilities.

At the Sports Center, visitors can play tennis or mini-golf, play in a game room, or rent bikes.

Visitors may swim in the five-acre-lake, equipped with giant water slides, or just sunbathe on the beach. Fishing is allowed in the stocked lake from mid-March through October.

The antebellum plantation complex includes nineteen restored and authentically decorated buildings that came from their original sites throughout Georgia, giving a realistic look at life in the 1840s. A gristmill, a sorghum mill, a cider press, and an authentic bridge re-create the plantation days in Georgia. Beginning at 4:00 P.M., free tram rides leave every twenty minutes from the Welcome Center and Plantation. The Sunset Plantation Tour costs extra.

Confederate Hall shows "The War in Georgia," a multimedia exhibit of photos and a lighted map, and has an accompanying narration. Visitors see the battles of Atlanta and troop movements of Sherman's March to the Sea.

The exhibits at the Stone Mountain Museum highlight the people, stores, and activities that make the mountain a legend.

Zoo Atlanta's twenty-two-acre Wildlife Preserve and Petting Farm gives an up-close look at more than forty different species of animals in a natural setting. The Naturalist's Cabin houses snakes from the Southeast region. The Trader's Camp petting farm includes miniature horses, sheep, and pot-bellied pigs. The majority of the animals here have been injured or orphaned, making them unable to return to the wild. Many are, or were, native to Georgia.

Two Easter sunrise services, one held at the top and one held at the base of the mountain, begin at 7:45 A.M. on Easter Sunday annually.

You might like to spend the night at the park to give you more time to enjoy all the park offers. Guest rooms are available at the Evergreen Conference Center and the Stone Mountain Park Inn. The campground has 400 wooded lakeside sites, as well as a supply store. Limited reservations are accepted, subject to availability. You may stay a maximum of two weeks at the campground.

The Walk

The self-guided Nature Gardens Trail forms a ¾-mile loop through a forested area. Interpretive markers describe the unusual vegetation and geology of the area. You will see the most color in spring and fall in the gardens; in summer, you will find lush greenery.

Drive 0.7 mile straight past the West Gate entrance, Confederate Hall, and the greenhouse on Robert E. Lee Boulevard. Park in the lot opposite the entrance to the garden.

➤As you cross the road, look to the left of the entrance at the large big-leaf magnolia tree. The magnolia, though rare in Georgia, is common in the park. A created rock quarry greets you as you enter the garden.

➤Pick up a map and brochures at the kiosk. You will see signage for plants that are unique here.

➤Turn left at the kiosk and follow the path. Look for green arrows to keep you on the trail. You will be walking through the lush understory—everything that grows beneath the tree canopy—of an old hardwood forest in a creek bottom. The larger trees are more than one hundred years old. As you pass through a collection of more than 600 cultivated (non-native) azaleas, look for ferns and for English ivy, which is not native to the area.

When you reach the bridge, you have reached the end of the 1960s garden. The gardens beyond this point have been developed since then.

➤Turn right across the bridge. The stream below originates from rainwater that comes off the slopes of Stone Mountain.

A white oak on the left, felled by a storm, is a good indicator of the size of some of the mighty trees in the forest. Look to the left across the oak tree to see a shady glade planted exclusively with ferns. In the sunny glade on the right, other types of plants flourish with the ferns.

➤As you bear right, you will see a tulip poplar tree on the right and an American beech on the left. Both are among the largest of their kind in the forest. As you continue, you will come across several sweet gum trees. They are giants of the Eastern deciduous trees (trees that lose their leaves) in the forest.

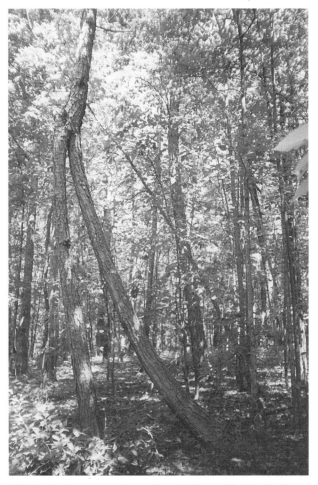

This fascinating tree can be seen from the Nature Gardens Trail.

➤Walk up the slope. Bear right at the marker at the top of the hill. Cross an ephemeral stream—one that flows according to rainfall—with moss-covered rocks.

➤Turn right at the marker at the top of the hill; then go downhill. On the left you will see the largest tulip poplar in the forest, perhaps 150 years old, and a big-leaf magnolia. On the right you will see the largest American beech in the garden. American beeches help determine the age of a forest, since they were one of the last of the hardwoods to come in. A beech this size indicates that the forest has been undisturbed since the tree was young.

➤Walk beside the winding creek. You will cross a stepping-stone granite bridge. On the left is a rock outcropping with an emerging underground spring that may be dry in summer.

As you walk uphill, on the right you will see mountain laurel, which flowers in spring. Usually this grows farther north, but the mountain protects the garden from summer heat, making a cool habitat. On the left you will pass a natural bench of large boulders.

➤Continue uphill. The overlook on the right offers a view of a different stream, which joins the first one farther down the hill. The water has worn the stones smooth over the years. You will pass yellow daisies, one of the native plants in the park. The daisies bloom abundantly the first two weeks in September.

As you continue uphill, you will see more stones as they emerge from the more shallow soil. Here the plant life changes: The trees do not grow as large as they do lower down, and more drought-tolerant plants grow there.

➤Turn right at the marker at the top of the hill. On the right you will see a chestnut oak, a tree that does not grow

Of Interest

The Making of a Carving

In 1916 the United Daughters of the Confederacy (UDC) bought the steep side of Stone Mountain for a Confederate memorial. Gutzon Borglum, sculptor, started the first carving showing Confederate generals Robert E. Lee and Stonewall Jackson and Pres. Jefferson Davis. The generals were on horseback and leading a 200-foot-high march of men, guns, and horses. The work stopped during World War I but resumed in 1922. In 1924 the UDC unveiled Lee's head, but again the project stopped. Borglum was dismissed following a disagreement with the UDC and later carved the famous giant sculpture of four U.S. presidents on the side of Mount Rushmore in South Dakota.

Augustus Lukeman took over the carving. In 1928 Lukeman unveiled Lee and his horse, Traveller, but quit in 1930 due to lack of money.

Time and the weather eroded the unfinished figures. Sculptor Walter Hancock started new work in 1963, completing the memorial in 1970.

in bottom land. It is hardier and can survive up higher, where it has less protection from the elements.

►Bear right as you go uphill; then go straight across a stream that has much exposed rock. The stream might be impassable for a short time after a storm.

You might see dead trees along the way that remain standing. Such trees play a part in a forest's ecology, becoming hollow—where birds can build nests inside. Insects infest the rotting wood, which draws woodpeckers. Mosses and lichens grow on rotting wood. Unless a dead tree endangers people, forest keepers allow it to stand.

Of Interest

Other Walks

The 1.3-mile trail—marked with yellow blazes—goes from the western base of the mountain to the summit. The elevation rises 800 feet in just a little more than a mile, and you will encounter some steep sections near the summit. You need to be in good physical condition and wear walking shoes or boots. Metal handrails assist walkers on those sections. The trail has a rest area with water at the halfway point. Do not pick any flowers on the trail. Visitors may not take domestic animals or bikes, nor may they litter, paint, or carve on the walk.

The strenuous 5-mile Cherokee Trail, with white blazes, encircles the mountain. You may begin this walk at Memorial Hall or start it at several other locations.

The 5-mile Robert E. Lee Boulevard provides a less strenuous way to walk around the mountain on sidewalks.

The park charges extra for the 1-mile Wildlife Trail. You will see animals and birds from different parts of the world in a natural forest habitat. Children enjoy the petting zoo.

➤Cross the bridge. You will pass a picnic table as you return to the entrance. On the right you will see a blend of native and cultivated azaleas.

Walk 17

Kennesaw National Battlefield Park

  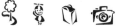

General location: This 2,864 park, steeped in Civil War history, is about 25 miles northwest of downtown Atlanta.

Special attractions: The park protects and preserves portions of Kennesaw Mountain and commemorates the entire 1864 Civil War campaign. It has 11 miles of Civil War earthworks, 16 miles of walking trails, and two open-air picnic areas.

Difficulty rating: Steep, with opportunities for sitting on rocks to rest. This walk takes you up the 650-foot-high mountain, 1,808 feet above sea level. You need to be in good shape for the trek, and you also need to wear sturdy walking shoes. The park has other walks on level ground. Ask for a map at the Visitor Center.

Kennesaw National Battlefield Park

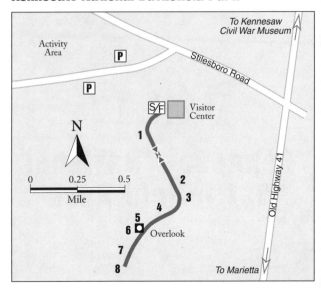

Distance: 2 miles, 1 mile up the mountain and 1 down. You may either walk down or take a bus down, or you may take a bus both ways. The view from the top of the mountain toward downtown Atlanta is well worth a look.

For those who feel up to walking 5 miles, get a map at the Visitor Center for the Little Kennesaw-Piegon Hill Loop. The Kennesaw-Cheatham Hill Loop covers 10 miles. Civil War buffs who are especially fit might want to get a trail map and hike the 16-mile loop to the Kolb Farm and back. This trek goes over the ground where the Confederate soldiers fought.

Estimated time: 1 to 1½ hours.

Walk 17

Services: The Visitor Center provides rest rooms, picnic tables, and grills. There is also a museum, a theater showing a twenty-minute film, and a gift shop and bookstore. Shuttle-bus to top of mountain is free. There are designated areas for picnicking, playing ball, flying kites, and for family fun. No admission is charged.

Restrictions: Do not walk or climb on fences or walk behind them. Dogs must be on leashes no longer than 6 feet, and owners must pick up "mutt mitts" at the headquarters or in the parking lots to pick up droppings off the trail and throw them into the woods. Visitors may not bring alcoholic beverages on the grounds. There is no bike riding on the trails, but horses are allowed on some trails. Visitors may park horses at the Cheatham Hill Road Visitor Center. Ask for directions for use of the three recreation fields. Stay off other fields. Start fires only in picnic grills. Picnic areas cannot be reserved. No camping.

For more information: Call Kennesaw National Battlefield Park.

Getting started: To reach the park from I–75 North, take exit 269 and turn left at the foot of the ramp onto Barrett Parkway. Go 2.1 miles and turn left onto Highway Old 41. Go 1.2 miles and turn right onto Stilesboro Road. Turn left into the park. You may park in the parking lot or in marked spaces on Highway Old 41.

Public transportation: None.

Overview: This park, a unit of the National Park Service, has the third-highest number of visitors to any historic site in the United States. In 1998, 1.2 million visitors from all fifty states and many foreign countries toured the park.

Try to take some time to walk around the park grounds, where so many men fought and died during the battles that took place there. Perhaps one of your ancestors fought at Kennesaw Mountain.

In the late spring of 1864, Union Gen. William T. Sherman left Chattanooga with an army of 100,000 men. His opponent, Confederate Gen. Joseph E. Johnston, left winter quarters at Dalton, Georgia, to oppose the Union troops with an army of 85,000. As he advanced, Sherman repeatedly feigned attacks on the Confederate forces while attempting to outflank and trap the Confederate forces, but Johnston always found a way to slip out of the trap. Sherman decided to slug it out with Johnston at Kennesaw Mountain.

On June 19 Johnston's Confederates entrenched themselves along the ridge tops of Big and Little Kennesaw Mountain south to the Powder Springs Road, blocking Union movement.

Sherman attacked Cheatham Hill and Pigeon Hill—two points in the Confederate position he felt were vulnerable. The unsuccessful attack produced 3,000 casualties as the Confederates held their earthworks, and Union soldiers nicknamed the place the "Dead Angle."

Checked by the Confederates, Sherman returned to his flanking maneuvers and continued his drive toward Atlanta. Sherman sent his forces southward, where they crossed the Chattahoochee River. After a lengthy siege Atlanta fell to the Union Army on September 2, 1864. The fall of Atlanta ensured Lincoln's reelection.

The Kennesaw Mountain National Park preserves the battleground where Johnston's army temporarily stopped the Union advance. Preserved here are the trenches largely responsible for the fleeting Southern victory.

The Walk

►Start at the Visitor Center. You will find markers along the way that tell about the Civil War. Always stay on the official trail and avoid shortcuts. Side trips can damage earthworks and the mountain terrain.

Of Interest

The Park's History

In 1914 a group of Illinois veterans purchased sixty acres around Cheatham Hill and built a monument honoring the Illinois brigade who had fought Confederate soldiers in the Battle of Kennesaw Mountain. The monument became the nucleus of the Kennesaw Mountain National Battlefield Park, and the War Department preserved it in the early twentieth century. The National Park Service bought the land for the park during the Great Depression in the 1930s for about $150,000. The present land value would reach into the billions of dollars.

The park opened August 10, 1933, after the Civilian Conservation Corps had developed it for several years. On June 27, 1964, the park dedicated a new center on the 100th anniversary of the Battle of Kennesaw Mountain. On the 130th anniversary of the battle in 1994, 6,000 visitors came that day alone. The unforeseen number of visitors prompted the move to add to the center.

The park underwent a $2.1-million expansion prior to the 135th anniversary in 1999. Visitors can see a movie about the battle in a video room and visit the bookstore, museum, library, and archives. The museum has three rare Confederate-made cannons, including one that had service during the battle.

►The first marker points out rifle pits—called "pickets"—Confederate soldiers used. Pickets were soldiers who went to the front of the line, alerting the main army of an attack. The 1st Alabama stopped the Union assault on this portion of the line at these pits. In battle often one side would capture the pits, and then the other side would recapture them.

►When you reach the marker that says .2 MILES TO THE TOP, follow the trail to the right. Along the way you might see a spring. Some springs appear only after a rainstorm, but a few flow all the time. Both Union and Confederate soldiers filled their canteens from these springs. Spring water was safer then than it is now, so please do not drink the water.

Although soldiers brought much food with them in their knapsacks, they still foraged for food in the woods. They found persimmons, sumac for "Indian lemonade," blackberries, hickory nuts, and chestnuts. These foods provided vitamins and nutrients, something absent in their military food rations.

►The third marker brings you to a historic road that settlers cleared before the war. This road cut across the wide trail on which you are now walking. If you look very carefully up the mountain, you can see this historic road. You can also see this road from different vantage points on the mountain. The Confederate soldiers hauled their cannons up this road, which served mainly for the movement of supplies and equipment during the battle.

►The fourth marker points out a Confederate trenchline, or earthwork, going uphill. Also, you can see another shortcut going uphill. Remember: Please do not use it; stay on the trail. The army used earthworks to provide cover while shooting at oncoming Union troops. This park has some of the most complex and extensive trenchlines constructed during the Civil War. Soldiers used shovels, picks, mess kits, and even their hands when digging them. You cross over them six times as you go up the mountain, so keep looking for them. You will then walk on a wooden walkway that protects the earthworks.

Going up the trail, you will see several types of trees, among them the cedar. The cedar has thin leaves, like pine needles; rough, flaky bark; and purplish, round fruit. A peach orchard stood on the mountain in the past.

As you approach the parking lot, you will see clusters of Japanese honeysuckle bushes on the right side of the trail. Its white and yellow flowers have a sweet smell and yield a thick, sweet liquid. On the down side, however, as a plant not native to the United States, it squeezes out native plants.

➤Marker 5 brings you to a historic overlook. Before the Civil War Marietta residents held picnics here to enjoy the view. From this position on the mountain, horses could no longer haul cannons, so soldiers had to haul the guns to the crest themselves!

➤Climb the steps to Marker 6, the Georgia overlook. This platform was built in 1964, one hundred years after the battle. A plaque on the front of this stone structure honors the fourteen Georgia Confederate generals who commanded troops during the Civil War.

➤Continue walking up the trail. Please stay off the earthworks in front of the gun emplacements. Notice the red oaks on both sides of the trail.

➤Marker 7 brings you to one of the four remaining emplacement fortifications. Confederate cannoneers dug these into the ground to protect them from the Union

Of Interest

Kennesaw Civil War Museum

As you leave the park, turn right onto Stilesboro Road, then left onto Highway 41. Cross Barrett Parkway, Cobb Parkway, and McCollum Drive. When you reach the second light, turn right across the railroad tracks and then turn left into the museum, located in an old cotton gin.

You are now in the town of Kennesaw, the starting point for the Great Locomotive Chase. A group of Union soldiers in civilian clothing, led by James J. Andrews, hijacked the train engine, the *General*, in an attempt to strike against the railroads of the South. You can read about the *Texas*, which pursued the *General*, in Walk 5. You can also visit the hotel where the raiders spent the night before the hijacking in Marietta, described in Walk 18.

The museum opened in 1972, almost 110 years after the Great Chase. Civil War memorabilia, including uniforms and firearms, a tattered Confederate flag, along with displays showing the importance of music during the war, are among the collection.

army that fired on them from below. As you continue, you will pass the remaining three earthen fortifications. The Napoleon cannons placed in these fortifications weighed about 1,300 pounds each. Horses could not be used at this terrain, so soldiers moved the cannons themselves.

Notice the large rocks on both sides of the trail, thought to date from the Lower Paleozoic era, about 300 million years ago. Called gneiss, this rock comes from quarries northwest of the park. Notice the lichen growing on the rocks and notice the red oak trees.

Walk 17

➤Marker 8 bring you to the signal platform. Both the Union and Confederate armies occupied the mountain at one time or another during the Civil War. When one army had control, it used this earthen structure as a signal platform. The armies sent flag—or "wig wag"—markers from the top of the mountain.

➤Retrace your steps to the end of the walk.

Walk 18

Historic Marietta

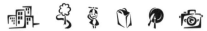

General location: Explore a historic town 17 miles north of Atlanta or 2.6 miles from National Battlefield Park, which you can read about in Walk 17.

Special attractions: Antebellum homes, charming restored historic square, and shops.

Difficulty rating: Easy; all on sidewalks on level ground; all paved.

Distance: 1.7 miles.

Estimated time: 50 minutes.

Services: Restaurants are located throughout town; rest rooms are available at Welcome Center.

Restrictions: Dogs must be on leashes no longer than 6 feet, and their droppings must be picked up.

Historic Marietta

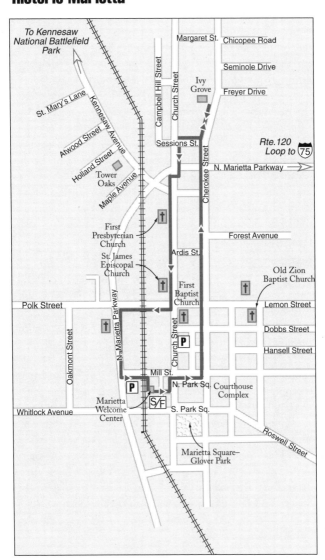

For more information: Contact the Marietta Welcome Center.

Getting started: The walk starts at the Marietta Welcome Center. Take Highway I–75 North to exit 265. Turn left and go 2 miles until you go through a light at Polk Street. On the left you will see the circa 1840 Virginia Plain plantation Root House, one of Marietta's oldest residences. Take the next left onto Mill Street; then turn right into the free parking lot. Walk across the railroad track on Mill; then turn right on the brick sidewalk. Enter the Welcome Center in the 1898 brick Western & Atlantic passenger depot, typical of passenger depots built at the turn of the century. This one replaced the 1840s depot that Sherman's army burned. The center offers a Marietta video, historic exhibits, and brochures about local events. You can pick up a map of an extended walking tour of the town.

Public transportation: None.

Overview: The Georgia legislature created Marietta in 1834, but no one knows how the town got its name. Probably it honors Mary Cobb, wife of Sen. Thomas W. Cobb, from whom the county gets its name. During the 1830s and 1840s, the Western & Atlantic Railroad came through, adding to the town's development.

Nineteenth-century Marietta became a resort. Its mild summers at 1,100 feet above sea level attracted planters escaping from the coastal heat and malarial swamps. After the Civil War Northerners joined Southerners there.

Three wars have influenced Marietta's development: the Civil War, World War II, and the Korean War. In 1864 Gen. William T. Sherman passed through the town, burning the courthouse and businesses around the square. (You may read about the battle at nearby Kennesaw Mountain in Walk 16.) Marietta recovered slowly, along with the rest of the South, after the Civil War. By 1900, however, the economy had recovered.

World War II brought the Bell Aircraft Company, which built a bomber plant here, giving the town its first major industry. Newcomers poured in to work at the plant. In 1945 Bell closed its doors, but in 1950 the Korean War brought the Lockheed-Georgia Company into the Bell facilities. During the 1950s and 1960s, it employed the largest number of people of any company in Georgia.

The present square and surrounding shops look as they did during the late nineteenth century.

Now enjoy a walk in an area rich in history through National Register Historic Districts.

The Walk

►Exit the Welcome Center through the door you entered and turn left onto the brick walkway. On the right you will see the 1850 Kennesaw House, which served first as a hotel in the town's early days. In 1864 it served as a Confederate hospital, and General Sherman had his headquarters there briefly.

The second floor houses the Marietta Museum of History, which contains artifacts from the early 1830s, when settlers and gold prospectors moved in after the government forced the Creek and Cherokee Indians off the land. It also houses an extensive textile collection of quilts, clothing, and needlework from circa 1810 to the present. James J. Andrews spent the night before he and twenty other spies hijacked the locomotive *General*, beginning the "Great Locomotive Chase" there. You may see the *General* at the Kennesaw Civil War Museum, mentioned in Walk 16.

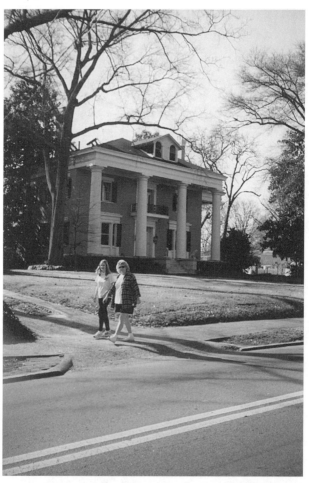

An impressive number of antebellum mansions are in Historic Marietta.

Walk 18

➤Walk the brick walkway straight ahead to the Marietta Square/Glover Park. Marietta's first mayor donated the land to the city around 1852.

➤Turn left on Church Street. You will pass the circa 1875 Brumby Chair Company. The company handcrafted its first rocking chair—thought to be Georgia's oldest product—just after the Civil War.

➤At the corner cross Church and walk beside the square on North Park Square.

➤Turn left at the corner onto Cherokee Street and cross North Park Square.

➤Cross Hansell, Dobbs, and Lemon Streets. Look to the right down Lemon to see the black Zion Baptist Church. Its new building is on the left, and the original building (circa 1866) is farther down on the right corner. Blacks built it shortly after the Civil War, when they formed their own church separate from the white church at the corner of Cherokee and Lemon Streets.

You are now entering an area where nearly every house is more than one hundred years old. Look for date markers on houses that are not mentioned in this guide.

➤Cross Ardis Street. Miss Virginia Crosby, descendant of George Washington's sister, lived in the 1888 house at number 201. She organized the Society of the Descendants of George Washington at a meeting in this house. She also had the distinction of being the first woman to run for mayor of Marietta.

Across the street at number 200, three sisters operated a boardinghouse in the 1890s, hosting guests who visited Marietta as a resort. Marietta had several popular boardinghouses such as this, with excellent meals and service.

You will pass an 1895 house at number 239.

➤Cross Kennesaw Avenue and North Marietta Parkway. Around 1870 a Confederate veteran first built a small house at number 362. As the area recovered from the effects of the Civil War and Reconstruction, his son enlarged the home to its present size.

➤Cross Sessions Street. A physician who bought the 1904 house at number 393 in 1922 renovated it to its present lovely condition.

A father built the circa 1895 house at number 403 as a wedding present for his daughter. The daughter and her husband later owned Ivy Grove, which you will see farther up the street.

Across the street at number 392, built around 1890, you will see an example of a house with classic Victorian lines.

The prestigious Atlanta architect Neel Reid designed the Georgian Revival home at number 419 for Otis A. Brumby, Sr., who published two newspapers.

You will come to Ivy Grove, a house built around 1843 on an estate that originally contained 1,800 acres. Edward Denmead, one of the town's pioneer settlers and mayor for eleven successive terms, built it. The family lost much of their fortune as a result of the Civil War and had to sell Ivy Grove in 1874. The house has undergone several restorations and remodelings.

➤Retrace your steps and turn right on Sessions Street.

➤Turn left on Church Street. You will pass an 1895 Greek Revival house at number 331 that reflects the heritage of antebellum grandeur.

➤When you reach the corner of Sessions and North Marietta Parkway, look across to the right to see Brumby Lofts, apartments that now occupy the old Brumby Chair Factory.

Walk 18

➤Cross North Marietta Parkway.

➤Turn right, cross at the crosswalk, and then turn left.

The Presbyterian Church built the house at 262 Church Street in 1849 for its ministers, who lived there over a period of more than one hundred years.

➤If you have limited time, continue straight on Church Street at this point. Otherwise, cross Kennesaw Avenue, turn right, cross the railroad tracks, and walk 0.6 mile on Kennesaw Avenue to see more historic houses.

After crossing the tracks, you will come to 243 Kennesaw, on the left. The original owners built it around 1840, during the first boom of frame construction in the early history of the town. This is an example of a Plantation Plain–style home, with a typical four-room arrangement. Its Victorian appearance is a result of remodeling.

➤Cross Maple Avenue. You will pass a circa 1883 Victorian-style house at the corner. Thomas M. Brumby of the Brumby Chair Company family bought the house, which was originally built by a prosperous merchant.

Look across the street to see the circa 1901 charming Victorian cottage-style house behind the white picket fence at number 264. A foreman of the Brumby Chair Company later owned the house.

James Brumby, founder of the Brumby Chair Company, supervised the building of Tower Oaks, at number 285, around 1882. An 1885 drawing shows that the house still has its original external appearance. The descendants of a judge who bought the house in 1922 still live there.

The next house shows a beautiful Victorian-style house, typical of those built in the nineteenth century.

You will next pass the classic 1843 Greek Revival house, which has the second largest Doric columns on a private house in Georgia. The columns are more than 11 feet in circumference at the base. Granite slabs for the porch and front steps were hauled from Stone Mountain by oxcart in 1865. A Union officer who headquartered here during the Civil War provided food for the starving local residents after the war. The house later served as a girls' seminary.

➤Cross Holland Street. Across the street at number 354 you will see the circa 1850 childhood home of Alice McClellan Birney, founder of the National Parent-Teacher Association. An 1985 move brought it here from its original location on Church Street.

➤At the corner of Kennesaw Avenue and Atwood Street, look ahead to see Tranquilla, a Greek Revival structure built in 1849 by General Andrew J. Hansell. The Hansell family occupied the house between 1849 and 1867. During the Civil War the house was occupied by Union officers, who inflicted much damage. Mrs. Hansell, who refused to leave, prevented more damage from occurring.

➤Retrace your steps to Church Street and turn right.

Woodrow Wilson's aunt had the Victorian-style Stanley House across the street built as a summer cottage around 1895.

The circa 1882 house at number 228 has always remained in the same family.

The house at number 218, built around 1890, started as a two-story Victorian. Remodeling turned it into a Georgian style after a 1925 fire.

The main section of the house at number 212—originally a story-and-a-half "shotgun" house—was built before the Civil War. A shotgun house got its name from the fact that a person could fire a gun at the front door and the shot would pass through the rooms lined up one behind the other. In 1929 the owner added a second story. Long used as a boardinghouse, it became famous for its Sunday dinners.

The circa 1855 house at number 202—remodeled as an insurance office—shows a beautiful example of adaptable restoration.

The Marlow House at number 192, built around 1887, served as a boardinghouse for forty-two years and now hosts weddings and other special events.

You will pass the First Presbyterian Church, organized in 1854. The Union Army used the 1854 Greek classic–style building as a hospital during the Civil War. A mixture of Georgia red clay and buttermilk made up original paint on the inside walls. The church had a gallery where slaves could worship.

The St. James Episcopal Church next door, originally built in 1843, burned in 1964. The military commandeered the facilities during the Civil War.

The octagonal-style building across the street opened in 1893 as the town's first library. Sarah Freeman Clarke, who had established a lending library in her home, raised money for a permanent structure. Today the building houses an art museum.

Across the street you will see the First Baptist Church, organized in 1835. The 1892 chapel, made of Georgia granite and marble, reflects both Gothic and Roman architecture.

➤Cross Polk Street; then turn right. Behind the Episcopal Church you will see a small portion of the 1878 structure that the church now uses as a chapel. The chapel houses an organ—which sat in the original sanctuary—that the Union troops filled with molasses during the Civil War.

➤At the bottom of the hill, turn left on N. Marietta Parkway. The Root House sits on the corner. You will experience the life of a middle-class merchant in this restored plantation-style home. In 1845 William Root, a pharmacist from Philadelphia, and his wife, Hannah, built this house, which is now decorated with authentic period pieces. Walk among the flower beds and vegetable plots, featuring only plants that were available in Cobb County before 1860. Root helped start St. James Episcopal Church.

➤Walk straight ahead, cross Mill Street, and return to the Welcome Center and the end of the walk.

Appendix A: Other Sights

You may enjoy several other attractions that are in or near Atlanta that tourists and local residents have enjoyed.

Gilbert House
2238 Perkerson Road, SW
Atlanta 30315
(404) 766–9049
This restored circa 1865 farmhouse has been called "Atlanta's Most Historic House." Call to find out when the house is open.

Hammonds House
503 Peeples Street, SE
Atlanta 30310
(404) 752–8730
Hammonds House is Atlanta's only African-American art museum.

Michael C. Carlos Museum
Emory University
571 S. Kilgo Street
Atlanta 30322
(404) 727–4282
This museum houses more than 16,000 ancient art objects from Egypt, Greece, Rome, the Near East, Asia, the Americas, Australia, and New Zealand. There is a $5.00 admission donation.

Scitrek
395 Piedmont Avenue
Atlanta 30308
(404) 522–3955 or (800) 524–6750
Georgia's high-tech playground offers kids hands-on exploration of science, mathematics, and technology. Admission is charged.

The William Bremen Jewish Heritage Museum
The Selig Center
1440 Spring Street, NW
Atlanta 30309
(404) 873–1661

Wren's Nest
1050 Gordon Street, SW
Atlanta 30310
(404) 753–8535
Wren's Nest is the home of Joel Chandler Harris, who wrote the Br'er Rabbit stories.

Appendix B: Contact Information

Throughout this book we have advised you to contact local attractions, museums, and shops to confirm opening times, locations, and entrance fees. Below are phone numbers and addresses of the places mentioned.

Apex Museum

135 Auburn Avenue

Atlanta 30303

(404) 521–2739

Atlanta Botanical Garden

1345 Piedmont Road, NE

Atlanta 30309

(404) 876–5859

Atlanta Convention and Visitors Bureau, Visitor Information Center

65 Upper Alabama Street

Atlanta 30303

(404) 521–6600; Out-of-state: (800) ATLANTA

www.atlanta.com

Atlanta Cyclorama

800 Cherokee Avenue, SE

Atlanta 30315

(404) 658–7625

Atlanta History Center

130 West Paces Ferry Road, NW

Atlanta 30305-1366

(404) 814–4000

www.atlhist.org

Atlanta Parks and Recreation Department

675 Ponce de Leon Avenue, NE

Atlanta 30308

(404) 817–6752

Atlanta Preservation Center Guided Walking Tours

537 Peachtree Street, NE

Atlanta 30308-2228

(404) 876–2040

Tours canceled in case of rain except for the Fox Theater tours.

Auburn Avenue Library and Research Center for African-American Culture & History

100 Auburn Avenue

Atlanta 30303

(404) 730–4001

Carter Presidential Center

441 Freedom Parkway

Atlanta 30307

(404) 331–0296

http://carterlibrary.galileo.peachnet.edu

Centennial Olympic Park

Marietta Street & Techwood Drive

Atlanta 30303

(404) 222–7275

Clark Atlanta University

223 James P. Brawley Drive, SW

Atlanta 30314

(404) 880–8000

CNN Center

247 CNN Center

Atlanta 30303

(404) 827–2300

Ebenezer Baptist Church

407 Auburn Avenue, NE

Atlanta 30312

(404) 688–7263

Emory University

1380 South Oxford Road, NE

Atlanta 30322

(404) 727–6123

www.emory.edu

Fernbank Museum of Natural History

767 Clifton Road, NE

Atlanta 30307

(404) 929–6300

Fernbank Science Center

156 Heaton Park Drive, NE

Atlanta 30307

(404) 378–4311

www.fernbank.edu

Fox Theater

660 Peachtree Street, NE

Atlanta 30309

(404) 249–6400

Georgia Institute of Technology
225 North Avenue, NW
Atlanta 30332
(404) 894–2000

Georgia State Capitol
206 Washington Street
Atlanta 30334
(404) 656–2844

Georgia State University
University Plaza
Atlanta 30303-3083
(404) 651–2000
www.gsu.edu

Governor's Mansion
391 West Paces Ferry Road
Atlanta 30305
(404) 261–1776

Herndon Home
587 University Place, NW
Atlanta 30314
(404) 581–9813

High Museum of Art
1280 Peachtree Street
Atlanta 30309
(404) 733–4444

High Museum of Art at the Georgia-Pacific Center
133 Peachtree Street
Atlanta 30303
(404) 577–6940

Historic Oakland Cemetery
248 Oakland Avenue, SE
Atlanta 30312
(404) 688–2107
www.oaklandcemetery.com

Interdenominational Theological Center
700 Martin Luther King Jr. Drive
Atlanta 30314
(404) 527-7700

Kennesaw Civil War Museum
2829 Cherokee Street
Kennesaw 30144
(770) 427–2117 or (800) 742–6897
www.nps.gov/kemo

Kennesaw National Battlefield Park
900 Kennesaw Mountain Drive
Kennesaw 30152
(770) 427–4686

Margaret Mitchell House & Museum
990 Peachtree Street, NE
Atlanta 30309
(404) 249–7015
www.gwtw.org

Marietta Welcome Center

4 Depot Street

Marietta 30060

(770) 429–1115 or (800) 835–0445

MARTA

(404) 848–4711

Martin Luther King Jr. Center for Nonviolent Social Change

449 Auburn Avenue, NE

Atlanta 30312

(404) 526–8923

Martin Luther King, Jr. National Historic Site, National Park Service Visitor Center

450 Auburn Avenue, NE

Atlanta 30312-1525

(404) 331–5198, ext. 3017

www.nps.gov/malu.

Morehouse College

830 Westview Drive, SW

Atlanta 30314

(404) 681-2800

Morehouse School of Medicine

720 Westview Drive

Atlanta 30310

(404) 752-1500

Morris Brown College
643 Martin Luther King Jr. Drive
Atlanta 30314
(404) 739–1000

Outdoor Activity Center
1442 Richland Road, SW
Atlanta 30310
(404) 752–5385

Piedmont Park
1085 Piedmont Avenue, NE
Atlanta 30309
(404) 875–7275
www.piedmontpark.org

Robert W. Woodruff Arts Center
1280 Peachtree Street
Atlanta 30309
(404) 892–2414

Root House Museum
Corner of North Marietta Loop and Polk Street
Marietta 30060
(770) 426–4982

Spelman College
350 Spelman Lane, SW
Atlanta 30314
(404) 681–3643

Stone Mountain Memorial Park

Highway 78

Stone Mountain 30086

(770) 498–5690 or (800) 317–2006

www.stonemountainpark.com

Trees Atlanta

96 Poplar Street, NW

Atlanta 30303

(404) 522–4097

www.treesatlanta.org

World of Coca-Cola Atlanta

55 Martin Luther King Jr. Drive

Atlanta 30303

(404) 676–5151

Zoo Atlanta

800 Cherokee Avenue

Atlanta 30315

(404) 624–5600

www.zooatlanta.org.

Appendix C: Read All about It

Want to read more about Atlanta, Marietta, Stone Mountain, and Georgia? The following books are but a sample of the many books you might enjoy.

Nonfiction

Buffington, Perry and Kim Underwood. *Archival Atlanta.* Atlanta: Peachtree Publishers, 1996. A humorous look at the city's history.

Davis, Ren and Helen. *Atlanta Walks,* 2nd Edition. Atlanta: Peachtree Publishers, Ltd., 1998.

Edwards, Anne. *Road to Tara: The Life of Margaret Mitchell.* N.Y.: Dell Publishing Co., Inc., 1983.

Eskridge, Jane. *Before Scarlett: Girlhood Writings of Margaret Mitchell.* Athens, Ga.: Hill Street Press, 2000.

Gourney, Isabelle, *AIA Guide to the Architecture of Atlanta.* Athens, Ga.: University of Georgia Press, 1993.

Simon, Jordan, and Jeff Clark. *Atlanta.* Marietta, Ga.: Longstreet Press, 1998. A detailed guide to eating, shopping, night life, and body building in the different sections of town.

The Swan's Palette. Atlanta: Forward Arts Foundation of Atlanta, 2000. Includes recipes served at the Swan Coach House tearoom on the campus of the Atlanta History Center.

Fiction

Mitchell, Margaret. *Gone With the Wind.* N.Y.: MacMillan (1936). The world's most famous novel.

Index

Meet the Author

Sara Hines Martin is a freelance writer living in suburban Atlanta. She grew up in Virginia, has lived in several states and in two third-world countries, and has visited a total of thirteen countries. She settled in Georgia twenty years ago and has gotten to know her adopted state in the same way she got to know the foreign countries in which she lived: exploring its geography, reading its history, and visiting its sites of interest.

She has been writing articles and books for forty-five years and now writes for several Georgia magazines and some national magazines for seniors. Her favorite recreation is walking, and she belongs to a hiking club that hikes in the mountains of North Georgia and North Alabama. She also loves history and enjoyed combining her two loves to get to know Atlanta, where she left no stone unturned in getting information for this book.

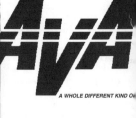
A WHOLE DIFFERENT KIND OF

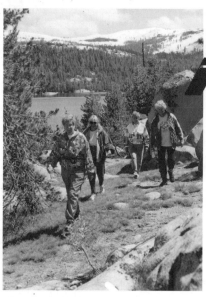

Experience A Whole Different Kind of Walk

The American Volkssport Association, America's premier walking organization, provides noncompetitive sporting events for outdoor enthusiasts. More than 500 volkssport (translated "sport of the people") clubs sponsor walks in scenic and historic areas nationwide. Earn special awards for your participation.

For a free general information packet, including a listing of clubs in your state, call 1-800-830-WALK (1-800-830-9255).

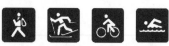

American Volkssport Association is a nonprofit, tax-exempt national organization dedicated to promoting the benefits health and physical fitness for people of all ages.